Notes of Encouragement

Reflections on the joy and power of practicing distinctively Christian healthcare

Paul O. Gerritson, MDiv

Christian Healthcare Insights
Durham, North Carolina

Published by Christian Healthcare Insights
3704 Sunningdale Way
Durham, NC 27707

ChristianHealthcareInsights@gmail.com

Ordering Information:

Quantity sales. Special discounts are available on quantity purchases by corporations, associations, and others. For details, contact the publisher at the address above.

Printed in the United States of America

First Printing, 2016

ISBN 978-0-9979154-0-2

Editing and Book Design by Margie Tippett

Major headings and text in Palatino
Article titles in Meiryo

Disclaimer

iii

Contents

Foreword

Since reading Dr. Gene Rudd's *Practice by the Book* (Bristol, Christian Medical & Dental Associations, 2005) several years ago, I have strived more intentionally to be a Christian doctor as opposed to being a doctor who just happens to be a Christian. As with many of you, it is my desire to proclaim the glories of Christ in my daily interactions with patients and staff as I pursue my calling as a physician and the practice of medicine.

Even with that desire and having felt this calling, I have struggled to keep Christ and the eternal as the focus of what I do minute to minute, hour to hour, and day to day. I am often sidetracked in this endeavor by the sheer number of tasks to be completed, the various boxes to be checked or clicked, phone calls to be answered, prior authorizations to be reviewed, and patients to be seen. It seems the more I struggle and become frustrated by ICD-10, EHRs, ACA, and meaningful use, the less focused I become on seeing my patients as weary travelers on the long journey of life in need of comfort, healing, encouragement, and a Savior. How do I keep my focus and make my practice of medicine eternally meaningful with the winds and waves of "progress" crashing all around distracting and discouraging me as I try to walk by faith and attempt to glorify Jesus by the work of my hands? How do I keep running the race to which God has called me– to be His ambassador of reconciliation – instead of becoming an apathetic and bitter physician?

I have struggled with these thoughts and feelings over the last several years as I have resisted the changes to the way I practice and care for my patients. I have become frustrated, angry, and bitter as I have felt powerless to protect what I perceive as a loss of the doctor-patient relationship. Frequently I have allowed these feelings to spill over and affect my relationship with friends, family, and even my God. Admittedly, I stepped out of the boat, started walking and then became fearful of the storm and started to sink. When I finally became desperate and called out to the One who can calm the waves, I was sent a friend and a brother to remind me that my life, my family, and my practice of medicine are built on a solid, unshakeable rock – the chief cornerstone – who is Christ Jesus. As I have been reminded to look upward to our Savior and inward to our source and strength, the Holy Spirit, I have been encouraged and energized to continue to strive daily to express God's love through the practice of medicine.

My friend and brother, Paul Gerritson, is this one sent by God to renew me. He has prayed for me, encouraged me, instructed me, admonished me, blessed me, and helped me to endure. Pastor Paul has been a great inspiration and motivated me to keep my gaze on Christ and more intentionally and consistently attempt to live out the gospel through the practice of medicine. I have been blessed by his fellowship and discipleship and am glad that he is now bringing to print many "healing leaves" of his inspiring words. I hope that they may bring healing and encouragement to many of my weary and frustrated brothers and sisters in the practice of healthcare.

Pastor Paul's life has uniquely qualified him to write this devotional to healthcare providers with excellence. He has worked in the healthcare arena and understands the pressures of providing high quality technical care during difficult and pressured situations while attempting to maintain compassion to sometimes hard to love patients. He has had to access and engage the medical community as a husband and caregiver of a dying wife. He has pastored physicians and dentists, coming alongside them to understand the many challenges and pressures we face as healthcare providers. Finally, in his study of the Word, God has granted him tremendous knowledge and skill in his application of scripture.

I am thankful to have him as a friend and pastor and hope that the Holy Spirit will use these writings to fill your cup as they have mine. Please read and cherish these words and let them remind you of your gracious God, His provision for your life, and his desire that you enjoy Him and glorify Him with your life and practice of medicine.

Zane Lapinskes, MD

Introduction

In 1992, God orchestrated my circumstances such that I came to put my faith in Jesus Christ as my Savior and Lord in the same year I was studying to become an EMT Basic. My first pastor, Larry Cox, taught me I had to read the Bible for myself, not just listen to the pastor's interpretations. So I began by reading all four Gospels, trying to learn more about Jesus. What I discovered has been the theme of my life ever since.

Jesus used excellence at healing bodies and teaching souls (emotions, intellect, memories, and will) to earn the attention and authority to speak to the spirits (the desire and capacity to commune with the Divine) of people. He gave that ability to the disciples with Him at the time. Today, Christians in healthcare are not superior to any other Christians in any other vocation, but they do have the privileged position of being the only people who can continue in the footsteps of Jesus by healing, teaching, and speaking all in a single patient encounter, as He did.

As a Critical Care Paramedic and Pastor, for more than two decades I've focused my life on teaching others how to exploit this privileged position for maximum kingdom growth, ministry, and glory to God. I equip healthcare ambassadors of reconciliation to faithfully sow seeds exposing the love and hope found in Jesus. Along the way, the Lord has allowed me to also help Christians in healthcare find rest for their souls, and renewed meaning and purpose in healthcare by restoring the sense that medicine is sacred ministry.

One tool I've successfully used to edify students and practitioners alike are these short teachings, called *Notes of Encouragement*. I'm amazed at the reader feedback detailing how they are equipped and emboldened to practice distinctively Christian healthcare. Occasionally, tears well up in their eyes as they ask, "How come nobody ever told me this before?"

May these Notes of Encouragement empower and inspire you, too! May you be drawn closer to Christ as you see yourself as His faithful servant, loving your neighbors daily, in His power, through the ministry of medicine. Rejoice! You'll discover you are a medical missionary right in your own community.

Pastor Paul

June 2016
Durham, North Carolina

CHRISTIAN HEALTHCARE

Is there such a thing as Christian healthcare?

If so, what is it that makes it distinctively Christian?

❧ What Is 'Christian Healthcare?'

Is there such a thing as "Christian healthcare?" This is a question commonly asked by Christians and non-Christians alike. You may ask this yourself. The answer is "Yes!"

One thing it is not is syncratically adding Christian features to the way you do healthcare. For example, being the kindest caregiver doesn't make it Christian healthcare; neither does wearing a crucifix around your neck or as a tattoo.

Going back to the Bible to see how Jesus cared for a person's body, soul, and spirit – often in the same encounter – is the foundation for defining Christian healthcare. Two themes which repeatedly appear in Christ's care are excellence at healing bodies and teaching souls, and then using that excellence as an authority-gaining platform for speaking of spiritual issues.

Though examples abound, Mark's account in Mark 4-6 of the healing of the legions-of-demons possessed man gives an outstanding example. In a single encounter, Jesus simultaneously dealt with the man's body, his soul, and his spiritual situation. He then directed him to reflect upon and witness to others the healing and redeeming works of God in his life. When the man publicly told what God had done for him and thus exposed Jesus, just as Jesus directed, entire communities were touched and healed. God got the glory. This account and many others lead to a definition which gets to the heart of the meaning of Christian healthcare:

> Exposing patients to Jesus while excellently
> healing bodies, teaching souls, speaking to spirits,
> *and* exuding the love, wisdom, and power of the Holy Spirit.

✑ One View of Christian Healthcare

We had the privilege of having a world-renowned Christian healthcare leader speak at one of our many student gatherings. What a gracious and humble servant and inspiration he was. We were blessed to hear his thoughts. For his evening presentation, he spoke on the *Marks of a Christian Physician*. I want to share briefly what I heard him share with us:

1. **Competency:** Are you practicing healthcare to the best of your ability? After all, we are to do everything as if we are serving the Lord. The attention of our patients and peers is earned through the quality of our care.

2. **Control:** Are you under the control of the flesh, acting selfishly, or under the control of the Holy Spirit, living sacrificially and humbly?

3. **Communication:** It is not enough to report facts to your patients or coworkers. We need to imbue our conversations with emotion and empathy, so that when we part ways, those who were with us will say, "My doctor understands me."

4. **Character:** Do we live a life of integrity such that those who know us trust us? Are we faithful in the small things?

5. **'Clones':** Are we reproducing disciples among those with whom we daily work, so they might expose Christ to others in what they say and do?

6. **Compassion:** We are hard pressed by our busy schedules, but do we use that as an excuse to ignore the humanity right before us or do we adopt an attitude like that of our Savior, who looked upon the myriad of hurting people as a flock that needed a shepherd?

What do you think about this definition? Given these marks, even if the Christian practitioner was exemplary according to these standards, how would our patients know Christ Jesus loves them, wants a relationship with them, and wants to be part of their lives now and forever?

Borrowing from Martin Luther on serving the Lord's Supper, without explaining in words what the sacrament means, bread and wine are little more than a communal snack service. In 1 Corinthians 14, Paul says our orderly, intelligible words explaining what people observe in our actions are essential attributes of Christ followers. These six marks may earn an attentive audience, but they aren't distinctively Christian in message. Without your voice, the actions alone are devoid of power to eternally transform.

ᕫ Is 'Nice' the Defining Distinctive?

Possibly the most asked question I hear from Christian healthcare students and practitioners is a variation on, "How can I be, remain, or show I am a Christian through my healthcare?" From the longest practicing to the newest students, the most often given response is a riff on, "Be nice" or "Be compassionate," followed quickly by, "Be competent," or "Be excellent, at what you do."

Upon reflection, such exchanges raise at least three challenging questions:

1. Should our main focus be showing we are Christ followers, or should it be to show forth Christ? (Being nice, compassionate, and competent certainly facilitates both efforts!)

2. If the defining distinctive of being a Christian healthcare practitioner is being compassionate and competent, then are we saying either almost all people in healthcare are Christians, or are we saying only Christians are capable of being authentically nice and practicing with excellence?

3. If we call ourselves Christians – followers and disciples of Christ Jesus – then what do we do with the not-very-nice bits of Jesus' example, like wielding a whip, overturning tables, declaring the powers of the day a 'brood of vipers,' or calling out Peter as an agent of Satan and a coward, etc.?

Space precludes a detailed discussion here, but a few brief principles ought to inform our thoughts and dialogue on the subject of being a practitioner of distinctively *Christian* healthcare.

Principle 1: Christians are His ambassadors (2 Corinthians 5:16-6:2) and are empowered by the Holy Spirit to be His witnesses (Acts 1:8). Our focus should be showing who He is, not who we are. That's called *exposing Jesus*.

Principle 2: While it is our mission as Christ followers to expose Him, it is never to *impose* Him. Not only is that professionally inappropriate but it is inconsistent with Jesus' own method of ministry.

Principle 3: We expose Jesus and avoid imposing Him when we salt our conversation as Jesus told the healed man to do: Tell what the Lord has done for us and about the loving mercy He has had on us (Mark 5:18-20). Give brief accounts of how God has met your physical or wisdom needs, and be ready to express how much God loved you by dying in your place and forgiving your sins.

Principle 4: We don't shy away from speaking to our peers and patients with gentleness and respect (1 Peter 3:14b-17) and speaking the truth in love (Ephesians 4:14-15) when we see their behavior is harmful or runs counter to the flourishing of themselves or others. We don't have to quote Bible verses at people, but we certainly can and should apply biblical principles to teaching souls, renewing minds, and thereby transforming lives. That's what Jesus did.

Nice is nice; it is arguably an essential for making straight the path for the Good News. However, it isn't a defining distinctive of Christian healthcare, for alone it doesn't point anyone to The One who truly heals and gives eternal life. Being and remaining a Christian healthcare practitioner means faithfully and fully serving through our vocation and voice as His witnesses and ambassadors, in His power and authority, according to His direction and model.

∂ What's Your Definition?

Often we speak of being a Christian healthcare practitioner. Is that a subjective term, or are there some recognizable benchmarks which can truly distinguish the Christian provider from all others?

Many great Christian practitioners have spoken or written on this question. We've heard them or read their works. They emphasize things like compassion and competence. They speak of our view of eternity, spirituality, values, priorities and relationships. In each of these words there is certainly a glimmer of God's Word and calling on every Christian's life, regardless of their vocation.

Let's not ever forget, though, that the distinctive of Christian healthcare is found in the Name itself – Christ, or Christ follower. Jesus Christ is the reason we think and act as we do. He's the reason we have a perspective that is distinctive from all others. In Jesus we find the comfort, love and power to touch the whole patient – body, soul and spirit. If it isn't Him we abide in, obey, and appropriately tell patients is the way to true healing, then it isn't Christian healthcare we render. It is a white-washed facsimile instead, merely making us look good and those around us feel good.

What's your definition of Christian healthcare? Have you ever tried to write it out? Live by it? Is it truly and distinctively Christian? Use this space to jot down your definition.

୶ New Creations & New Footsteps

I have often said, Christian healthcare practitioners are not superior Christians. However, since the work of our Heavenly Father that Jesus was doing in the world was healing (body), *and* teaching (soul: emotions, intellect, memories, and will) *and* speaking (midwifing and maturing the spirit), we can say that Christian healthcare practitioners have the greatest opportunity of all Christians to walk in Jesus' footsteps.

In light of the resurrection, here are two passages which speak on the power of the resurrection in the lives of believers. Since Jesus is alive, we as Christian healthcare practitioners are united with His life and living work ... the life and work of walking in Jesus' footsteps.

> *For we are of God's making, created in union with the Messiah Yeshua for a life of good actions already prepared by God for us to do.*
>
> Ephesians 2:10; Complete Jewish Bible

> *Therefore, if anyone is united with the Messiah, he is a new creation — the old has passed; look, what has come is fresh and new! And it is all from God, who through the Messiah has reconciled us to himself and has given us the work of that reconciliation, which is that God in the Messiah was reconciling mankind to himself, not counting their sins against them, and entrusting to us the message of reconciliation. Therefore, we are ambassadors of the Messiah; in effect, God is making his appeal through us. What we do is appeal on behalf of the Messiah, "Be reconciled to God!"*
>
> 2 Corinthians 5:17-20; CJB

I hope you spend at least a few minutes reflecting on this. There are millions of very skilled and competent practitioners in this world. They can participate in healing and teaching just as we can. There are also millions of Christians in this world who have all been saved through and into the risen Christ for the good work of appealing to the world to be reconciled with God. But you, beloved, are uniquely God's workmanship in your setting among your peers and patients. You can walk in the footsteps of Jesus. If you are listening to His call for you to do so, you can be certain, in and on His authority, that as His workmanship prepared for this work, He will be with you and equip you (Matthew 28:16-20; Acts 1:8). Together let's walk as He modeled for us to do.

⮦ Will This Too PAS?

The Move Toward Death on Demand

Christians are a curious lot. Collectively, we think about the death of our Savior every time we take the Lord's Supper. We think about getting to heaven after death, and look forward to the souls of the saints being reunited with resurrected bodies. When it comes to our own dying however, or that of loved ones or our patients, our theology seems thin. We default to following shifting cultural norms and our own desire for 'quality of life,' autonomy, and self-control as our guides for how to handle it. Thin theology and shallow thinking about dying have grave consequences – arguably they are tasteless salt, good for nothing but being trampled on and thrown on the manure pile.

> Thin theology and shallow thinking about dying have grave consequences.

In the last 100 years, we've begun reversing 2,500 years of healthcare history, starting when Greek followers of Hippocrates refused to actively kill anyone or refer to others to do it. Subsequently Christians throughout the Roman empire additionally cared for and thus gave dignity to the suffering until they passed away, and then gave them a respectable burial. The Hippocratic Oath, Bible-rooted compassion and valuing the sanctity of life, and the principle *Primum non nocere* (First, do no harm) have been hallmarks of the most advanced medical practices for centuries.

However, since 1930s Germany right up to today, under the disguises of 'compassion' and 'dignity,' as well as 'greatest-good economics,' societies are racing downhill toward the edge of a cliff, like so many demon-possessed pigs. Death,

death bobbing everywhere is their destiny as governments and practitioners around the world and across our nation pursue legalization of physician-assisted suicide (PAS). And in a strange twist of irony, the presumptively wise agents of death do not see that with the passage of PAS legislation (and the almost-certain subsequent 'civil right' to Death on Demand), medical servants will be transformed into slaves with no hope of escape to freedom except to quit medicine altogether. Not only physicians will be chained to this bizarre form of 'healthcare,' but so will nurses, physician assistants, and pharmacists, among others.

There is no question that end-of-life care through hospice and palliative care need educational, financial, legislative, and practitioner support. Christians in healthcare have a proud heritage in these arenas and each generation of practitioners has a duty to the great cloud of witnesses to continue advancing the relief of suffering and adding life to a person's remaining days.

However, improving the practice of relieving suffering shouldn't include killing sufferers as a solution. The Great Physician, Jesus, our role model for Christian healthcare, never – ever – resorted to killing as a solution to suffering, whether physical, mental, or spiritual. As His disciples, neither should we.

৯ Dr. King & 'Healthcare Injustice'

Reflecting on the life and work of Dr. Martin Luther King, Jr., I thought it might be good to look at one statement attributed to him about healthcare. "Of all the forms of inequality, injustice in health care is the most shocking and inhumane." As Amanda Moore has pointed out, however, nobody can seem to find a written or audio transcript of where or when Dr. King said this (http://www.huffingtonpost.com/amanda-moore/martin-luther-king-health-care_b_2506393.html). What she discovered was that it was apparently an extemporaneous remark that has been misquoted. An eyewitness to the statement, Dr. Quentin Young, said that Dr. King made the remark in conversation, not his presentation, at the 1966 convention of the Medical Committee for Human Rights. According to Dr. Young, the actual quote is, "Of all the forms of inequality, injustice in health care is the most shocking and inhuman."

The term "inhumane" implies broken humans are failing to care properly for other humans, while "inhuman" implies those causing healthcare injustice are not even human, but presumably something of a lesser species. The former, 'incorrect' statement condemns unjust *behavior*; the later 'correct' statement condemns the *people* who behave unjustly. Given what we know of Dr. King's heart, I presume he meant to say 'inhumane.'

> Our lives begin to end
>
> the day we become silent
>
> about things that matter.
>
> Dr. Martin Luther King

Our choice of words is some-thing to think about seriously as we engage with our patients, communities, and leaders about healthcare policy and access. It matters not only what our motives are, but also what and how we express our opinions. As Christians called to be salt and light, we really do need to be deliberately under the control of the Holy Spirit as we speak, so we can speak the truth in love boldly.

❧ A Christian's 'Charm Offensive'?

After years of political wrangling which never resolves anything but only keeps folks stirred up and anxious, we finally have something new from Washington, DC. The President of the United States is reportedly on a 'charm offensive.'

Regardless of your political persuasion, consider this for just a moment. There is something not quite right about a professing Christian having a huge media machine announce as news that the Christian is suddenly being 'charming.' Any Christian walking by the Spirit (Galatians 5:22-26) and who is maturing (2 Peter 1:5-8) should almost by definition be 'charming.' She or he should regularly be treating others with gentleness and respect. Charm ought to be self-evident and a daily state others can see readily, sans public proclamations from town criers.

How about us? Are the fruits of the Spirit and the marks of Christian maturity evident in our lives? Do those we study or practice with, regardless of their role in our organization, see us as 'charming?' Christian health care practitioners should not be seen by those around them as people who turn on charm as a means to an end, but authentic followers of Christ who consistently treat all people with gentleness and respect. Would our peers and patients believe us if we told them Jesus is renewing our minds, transforming our lives and conforming us to His image by the power of His Word and the Holy Spirit? Would they naturally call us 'charming' or would our becoming gentle and respectful be breaking news?

14

JESUS

If Christian healthcare is following Jesus' example,

then we ought to remind ourselves of

some things about Him.

☞ Alone!

Mark 14 has few equals in Scripture as a tangible example of the struggle between good and evil, light and darkness, and of spiritual warfare invading the affairs of humanity.

It replays the fall of mankind (Genesis 3-4) taken to an extreme. Along with Mark 15, it features the promised epic struggle in which the serpent will bruise the Messiah's heel, prior to the Messiah crushing the serpent's head. Mark records, in a sense, Satan recruiting an entire brood of vipers to attack Jesus the Lamb's heels: lies, denial, betrayal, shame, violence, darkness, rejection of God are all writ large. In the Garden of Gethsemane, once again man runs away naked (v.51-52). Nobody in this account is shown as trustworthy or a truly devoted follower of God. The sordid history of the fall of humanity is replayed in vivid detail.

No wonder then that Jesus felt the need to pray. But when He took Peter, James and John (future 'pillars of the church,' Galatians 2:9) with Him to do so, they, too, failed Him, for their spirits were willing but their flesh was weak. Nobody would stand with Jesus – everyone would scatter. Jesus would be abandoned by all mankind and by His Father. He stood alone. He fell down sweating drops of blood alone. He was hung upon a tree oozing rivulets of blood, alone. He was buried alone after being pierced in the heart – alone. No wonder He "began to be deeply distressed and horrified," saying His "soul is swallowed up in sorrow – to the point of death."

Him alone. That's ultimately the point, isn't it? Jesus alone, as the one and only fully human and fully God, was able to stand against such sin and trauma. He alone was appointed and able to bear the sins of the world upon Himself – to become sin for us. By virtue of those bleeding stripes He took

16

on our behalf, we no longer have to stand alone, naked before God, without excuse and bearing full responsibility for our sins. Jesus has done that for us. Him alone.

Decades later, the Apostle Paul, who at one time had a big beef with the value of Mark but later came to see him as necessary to his ministry (Acts 15; 2 Timothy 4), took the events of Mark 14-15 and made sense out of them. He expounded the purpose of Jesus' necessary aloneness. In Romans 3:9-4:8, Paul revealed Jesus' loneliness as meaningful and applicable not only to us today, but to the whole world for all time to come.

When you engage your peers, patients, friends and family over the coming weeks, prayerfully seek ways to rejoice publicly in what the Lord has done for you and the loving mercy He has had on you. Express how grateful you are that because Jesus alone was able to bear the penalty for your sin, you are joyful! Because God's Spirit indwells you, you never live alone but stand with Him forever.

For I am not ashamed of the
Gospel, because it is God's
power for salvation to everyone
who believes, first to the Jew,
and also to the Greek.

Romans 1:16

❧ Being 'In Christ'

As Christians in healthcare, there are at least three good reasons why being in Christ should be of interest to you. First, it reflects our being made in God's image and likeness to the world, including our patients. Second, as medical students and practitioners, we want to be able to give hope to those we minister to in body, soul and spirit, including how to live a fruitful life, no matter how short time on earth may be. Third, being in Christ brings with it a myriad of blessings. Let's explore each reason just a bit deeper.

Created by God in His image and likeness ... in Christ

Part of humans being created in God's image is each person having a desire for eternity or spiritual things. That aspect of reflecting God finds its fullest expression when we are born again – when God's Spirit indwells us so His Holy Spirit can commune with our newly animated spirit. The Apostle Paul gave at least two comments on being born again so that we may live fully in God's image in Christ. First, *Therefore, if anyone is in Christ, he is a new creation; old things have passed away, and look, new things have come.* (2 Corinthians 5:17) Second, *For we are His creation, created in Christ Jesus for good works, which God prepared ahead of time so that we should walk in them.* (Ephesians 2:10) Eternal life, hope, and purpose are only found as we are found in Christ.

Created in His image and likeness to live a fruitful life ... in Christ

Jesus' most detailed dissertation on what it means to be created in Him is found in the Gospel of John, chapters 14-16, the heart of which is 15:7-8, *If you remain in Me and my words remain in you, ask whatever you want and it will be done for you. My Father is glorified by this: that you produce much fruit and*

18

prove to be My disciples. These are the good works prepared in advance for us to do, as well as maturing in the fruits of the spirit.

Created in His image and likeness for myriad blessings … in Christ

- Those found remaining in Christ are called "faithful saints." (Ephesians 1:1)

- In Christ we have every spiritual blessing in the heavenlies. (Ephesians 1:3)

- All new creation will one day find complete unity in Him. (Ephesians 1:9-10)

- In Christ we discover the Father's grace and kindness to us. (Ephesians 2:7)

- Our lives have eternal meaning and purpose in Christ. (Ephesians 2:10)

- In Christ our redemption and reconciliation is paid for. (Ephesians 2:13)

- Jews and Gentiles are co-heirs of God's promises in Christ. (Ephesians 3:6)

- By the church in Christ, we glorify our Heavenly Father. (Ephesians 3:21)

- In Christ, head of the church, we live lives in God's likeness. (Ephesians 4:15)

- Where is truth found? In Christ Jesus, our Teacher. (Ephesians 4:21)

Application

Sometimes our lives get so busy, so stressful, or maybe even so mundane, we lose sight of where we are. Possibly your life is going great right now but you know a peer or patient who is despairing. Either way, it is good for each one of us to pause and reflect on the fact we have been saved, are saved, and will be saved in Christ. This is the firm foundation we stand on now and forever more, and is a foundation worth recommending to those we contact and about whom we care.

> I am the vine; you are the branches. The one who remains in Me and I in him produces much fruit, because you can do nothing without Me.
>
> John 15:5

⌒∾ By *His* Stripes We Are Healed

> *Then Jesus said to His disciples, "If anyone wants*
> *to come with Me, he must deny himself, take up*
> *his cross, and follow Me. For whoever wants to*
> *save his life will lose it, but whoever loses his life*
> *because of Me will find it. What will it benefit a*
> *man if he gains the whole world yet loses his life?*
> *Or what will a man give in exchange for his life?*
> *For the Son of Man is going to come with His an-*
> *gels in the glory of His father, and then He will*
> *reward each according to what he has done."*
>
> Matthew 16:24-27

Many of us study diligently and work very hard to care for our patients to the best of our abilities. We take pride in what we do. I just wonder though how many of us carry these character traits into our faith-walk with Jesus? Even if we don't readily recognize it, how many of us try to study and work our way into God's good graces, earning or keeping our salvation?

Jesus is not coming back in glory with the angels to pay wages that are due to us for our exemplary life! He is coming back to reward (not pay) us for only one thing: laying aside our self-sufficiency by accepting what Jesus did for us on the cross and then walking in the Spirit where God leads us.

Our Lord has gifted and called you. He may use your hard work to minister to those who suffer. Remember thought it is only by *His* stripes anyone is truly and eternally healed. So at least in this area, relax and rejoice. He has done the work. It is finished. Amen.

ᘒ Should I Stay or Should I Go?

In June, we see healthcare students moving home, moving up or moving out. Residents and fellows are arriving. Things are in a bit of healthy flux. Are you considering moving spiritually, or making a medical ministry move? Is your motivation right? Is your motivation driven, at least in part, by a sense that you are not seeing any spiritual fruit or reaping a harvest where you practice? You blame the soil where you work for being barren. You think grass will be greener when people appreciate your spiritual labor.

God sometimes lets people work all night long, in the darkness, catching zero fish, even though they are experts at fishing. His purpose is to bring us to the end of ourselves and our expertise.

Maybe that's true. But if we look at the calling of Peter into ministry by Jesus, we must at least explore the possibility that God sometimes lets people work all night long, in the darkness, catching zero fish, even though they are experts at fishing. His purpose is to bring us to the end of ourselves and our expertise. This is to force us to listen to God's unchanging commission and obey precisely when *we* are *sure* it is pointless and fruitless.

In Luke 5:1-11, when Peter's expertise gave way to obedience to put back out into the 'barren' waters and cast the net again, only then did three things happen: physically, a catch so large it nearly sank two boats; in his soul, a realization that his own expertise had, in a way, become a sin of pride; and, in his spirit, Peter was charged with a transforming passion to follow Christ as Master and Lord.

We know that in the hearts of most of you, you want to see Jesus glorified as Lord and Master. You want to see a spiritual harvest among your peers, coworkers and patients. Among a group this large and diverse, some of you are seeing rich catches while others are pulling up empty nets. For all of us, let's keep in mind that while we are called to be trained and prepared to give explanations for the hope we have, and to expose the love of Jesus to those around us wherever we go, we must go trusting in God's power and Spirit and not in our expertise. If Jesus has called you into your boat on the waters, don't doubt His calling. Act faithfully and in obedience. Don't beach your boat and move on to another work unless He tells you to. You might just miss out on your miraculous catch as a blessing for your persevering obedience.

❧ Grieving & Mourning Together

Some seasons are much more somber than others. This has been one of those seasons for our Christian healthcare family. Some of us have just lost a dear friend or colleague to disease. Others have lost a colleague or classmates to murder. Still others are pained by the conditions in which we find our patients.

We hurt because our finest ministrations to our patients and their friends and families seem to be inadequate. Having myself experienced violence, disease, disability unimaginable, and death unexplainable in my medical and pastoral career, my heart goes out to those of you who are grieving and mourning now. So I won't presume to heap pastoral platitudes on you and worsen your pain. I'll just share a couple of brief thoughts rooted in my own experiences as a survivor of grief and mourning.

Your grief and mourning are real and wouldn't exist if you didn't bear the image of God, and as a Christian, the compassion of Christ. Don't let anyone downplay it or try to cut it off before you are through it. Along those lines, yes, Scripture says all of us are to mourn with those who mourn. It doesn't say, "Fix them." The best way to help those who are in this season is to sit quietly with them, simply making your servant-availability known. Then follow through when asked for help.

At some point, you may ask God or others, "Why?" questions. Fools presume to be omnipotent and give a specific answer, thinking they know what God alone knows. However, there are some general questions we might help with, such as "Why do I grieve or mourn?"

Scripture tends to use "grieve" in the context of a loss or something held dear that was taken away because of sin or evil. The person or thing we loved and cherished is now gone because we live in a broken, fallen world. God grieves over sin and so do we, as people made in His image. It is this grief, or fear of it, which compels us to hope for heaven, where there will be no evil, sin or brokenness.

Mourning tends to address loss in general, irrespective of cause. God created us to live forever and for all things to flourish. Loss of that which is loved is not God's creative design; eternity and a flourishing multiplication are. Our pain in mourning may one day morph into a very real reminder that, despite our current circumstances, God was, is and forever will be good to those who lean on Him. He has a way today for us to be certain of a future that restores the losses that matter. That way is to put our faith in Him who was acquainted with grief and bore our sorrows – Jesus.

The Spirit of the Lord GOD is on Me,
because the LORD has anointed Me
to bring good news to the poor.
He has sent Me to heal the brokenhearted,
to proclaim liberty to the captives
and freedom to the prisoners;
to proclaim the year of the LORD's favor,
and the day of our God's vengeance;
to comfort all who mourn,
to provide for those who mourn in Zion;
to give them a crown of beauty instead of ashes,
festive oil instead of mourning,
and splendid clothes instead of despair.
And they will be called righteous trees,
planted by the LORD to glorify Him.

Isaiah 61:1-3
(Jesus identified with this passage in Luke 4:16-21)

25

✑ A Humble Report Card

This note of encouragement has roots in many Scriptures, the most important being Matthew 25:14-30. Please read it.

At a meeting of practitioners, a man I highly respect for his love of God and his humility raised a deep concern of his. His supervisor expected him to write his own annual evaluation. In his setting, annual evaluations are a big deal. They can make or break future responsibilities, promotions, and raises. To my friend however, writing his own evaluation seemed the height of hubris. Even if he were completely forthright and honest in his self-evaluation, he dreaded appearing arrogant or braggadocious. He feared more than anything it might harm his Christian witness to be pointing out all the things he had done well.

There are several key points to keep in mind when seeking a solution to this situation. Let's look at a few of them.

First, his supervisor has authority over him. He's not asking for anything sinful or illegal. So the task, challenging as it is, is one he should resolve to fulfill. Don't forget great people like Daniel and his three amigos, Malachi and Esther, and Nehemiah were just a few women and men who were placed under the authority of Gentiles who didn't always see things God's way. Yet these saints were faithful to serve and be accountable to those over them.

Second, remember people like Joseph. He went from obscure slavery to viceroy of Egypt, and saved untold millions of lives because of three character-revealing principles:

1. In all he did, he saw himself as serving and glorifying God;

2. He did everything to the best of his ability; and,

3. He was accountable, whether to Potiphar or Pharaoh.

Finally, look at the example of the servants given talents to invest for the master. The master gave the talents, expected them to be used to the best of each servant's ability, and he rightfully expected an accounting. In the parable, the master is mortal. We know though that our Master gives each of us all of our talents and resources. He, too, will ask of us an accounting.

So write your evaluation as if giving a humble report card to Jesus. Show Him you've used what He's given you wisely. Consider it practice for the future as you account for your privileged position practicing Christian healthcare.

⁊ Flesh & Blood in Common

At Christmas we celebrate God taking on flesh in the form of an infant. It is a beautiful mental image. But His birth has to have greater meaning than beautiful imagery or it becomes just one of so many births. Thousands of infants are born daily around the world. All of them will potentially suffer. Death will come to each one day.

What made Jesus' birth so unique was its purpose and person, best described in this uncommon but appropriate Christmas passage:

> *Now since the children have flesh and blood in common, Jesus also shared in these, so that through His death He might destroy the one holding the power of death—that is, the Devil— and free those who were held in slavery all their lives by the fear of death. For it is clear that He does not reach out to help angels, but to help Abraham's offspring. Therefore, He had to be like His brothers in every way, so that He could become a merciful and faithful high priest in service to God, to make propitiation for the sins of the people. For since He Himself was tested and has suffered, He is able to help those who are tested.*
>
> Hebrews 2:14-18

As you engage with those who are suffering, fearing death, or are realizing it will soon take them, keep this passage in mind. In sharing it with another person, you have the opportunity to bring forth the entire Gospel story. Hope can shine forth. Fear might be dispelled. A companion in suffering may be found. Eternal life may well be offered and claimed! These are enduring tidings of Good News!

The Holy Spirit

He is the greatest gift and power we possess.

Savor a small taste of what He wants to do through you.

⌘ Our Glorious Ministry

No matter how high or low you are in the pecking order of healthcare, no doubt you are seeing change. While patient autonomy gets lots of press and priority, the autonomy of the practitioners appears to be shrinking. Thus the frequent comments I hear about how what once seemed to be a glorious ministry of healing is becoming, in many aspects, a grind.

Through the prophet Haggai, God called His people not to focus on paneling their own estates. In Haggai 1:7-9, the people were told to get back to work building His temple in order to bring Him glory. The people obeyed, but their passion and strength were weak. The results of their work didn't seem to measure up to what they recalled from their past efforts. They obeyed but were disheartened.

> "Not by strength or by might, but by My Spirit," says the LORD of Hosts.
>
> Zechariah 4:6

So God came again to the people – all of them – regardless of their ranking and role. What He brought them was a hopeful message of encouragement. The message began like this:

> *On the twenty-first day of the seventh month, the word of the LORD came through Haggai the prophet: "Speak to Zerubbabel son of Shealtiel, governor of Judah, to the high priest Joshua son of Jehozadak, and to the remnant of the people: Who is left among you who saw this house in its former glory? How does it look to you now? Doesn't it seem like nothing to you? Even so, be strong, Zerubbabel"—this is the LORD's declaration. "Be*

strong, Joshua son of Jehozadak, high priest. Be strong, all you people of the land"—this is the LORD's declaration. "Work! For I am with you"— the declaration of the LORD of Hosts. "This is the promise I made to you when you came out of Egypt, and My Spirit is present among you; don't be afraid."

Haggai 2:1-5

God's Spirit is among us, too! The Holy Spirit indwells every follower of Jesus. Thus we are empowered to be His witnesses, His ambassadors of reconciliation, and His voice of love, grace, hope, and peace. We have the wisdom and words of God at our disposal. Medicine may not seem as grand as it once did. Its luster may have worn off. Our part seems small. But our God takes the small things like little faith and the mustard seeds of telling what the Lord has done for us and the loving mercy He's had on us and uses them to save souls who become new temples for the Holy Spirit, just as you are.

Be strong! Don't be afraid of the future! God is present with us in our healthcare ministry. We'll recognize Him and His work when we focus on using our temporary vocation of healthcare as a platform for fulfilling our eternal calling to bring God glory. In so doing, we'll see our grind become a glorious ministry once again.

ᘒ Overshadowed by God's Power

When reading Mark 8-9, the overarching lesson for those of us in Christian healthcare is that we need to develop our spiritual vision. We need to become people who not only see with our physical eyes, but grow to see things spiritually. That means seeing things the way God might see them. The past foreshadows the present. The present is not always what it appears. God's vision of the future of believers is always more amazing than we can imagine. Finally, we need to look at the internals – the soul and spirit – if we are going to really see renewal and transformation. Let's apply spiritual vision to the concept of God's overshadowing.

Mark 9:7 says this about the future apostles Peter, James, and John on the Mount of Transfiguration: *A cloud appeared, overshadowing them, and a voice came from the cloud: This is My beloved Son; listen to Him!* This concept of overshadowing isn't unique to Mark's Gospel, where the overshadowed three amigos began to be Apostles rather than merely followers of Jesus. We find overshadowing in Genesis 1:2 when God's Spirit overshadowed the formless and void earth, just before God began speaking His creative words of transfiguration. We find overshadowing again in Luke 1:34-35 when Mary asks Gabriel how a virgin could conceive and give birth to the Son of the Most High. The God-man would be created by the Holy Spirit's overshadowing.

> We need to become people who not only see with our physical eyes, but grow to see things spiritually. That means seeing things the way God might see them.

32

At least two New Testament passages allude to God using His followers as agents of His overshadowing power. One example is Acts 1:8. *But you will receive power when the Holy Spirit has come on you, and you will be My witnesses in Jerusalem, in all Judea and Samaria, and to the ends of the earth.* Or how about Peter, who had been overshadowed and received God's power, as an example, in Acts 5:12-16? *...As a result, they would carry the sick out into the streets and lay them on cots and mats so that when Peter came by, at least his shadow might fall on some of them...and they were all healed.*

In each case, overshadowing was followed by the peeling back of what was seen to reveal things unseen and amazing. New creation followed. Spiritual eyes were opened. For some, the spiritual eyes were opened immediately. Maybe our spiritual eyes are opened years later as we read the biblical accounts.

With this idea in mind, what should we make of the idea of God still at work overshadowing? How might thinking of God using His followers as agents of His overshadowing alter how we view our healthcare ministry?

When you enter the presence of a patient, delivering Christian healthcare means that you take the indwelling Holy Spirit with you. You go with access to God's overshadowing, transformational power. You have the power to be Jesus' witness as well as see God at work making a new creation. I invite you to read 2 Corinthians 5:13-21 and see if you can spiritually envision yourself an agent of God's overshadowing.

❧ Gifts to Tame Healthcare Tempests

Background: Mark 4:36-41 and Matthew 14:22-33

Healthcare is undergoing tempestuous change. As Christians in the wind and the waves of practice every day, you know the stormy secular and sacred issues that arise, sometimes fiercely. Our Lord Jesus doesn't want us rowing our careers futilely, in fear and in darkness. He sits on high watching and praying for us and has given us the gifts we need to travel over the waves and arrive safely at our shore.

The first gift for every Christian is the indwelling Holy Spirit. *The Father will give you another Counselor to be with you forever. He is the Spirit of Truth…He remains with you and will be in you…I will not leave you as orphans* (John 14:15-18). The Holy Spirit will remind us of all the things the Lord Jesus has said. Applying the truth of God's teachings and principles to how we conduct our lives is called wisdom. But, as James 5:1-8 says, when we ask the Holy Spirit for wisdom, we must act on what we hear – without doubt – or we will remain storm-tossed and unstable.

> **Our Lord Jesus doesn't want us rowing our careers futilely, in fear and in darkness.**

The second gift is God's written Word, the Bible (see 2 Timothy 3:16-17 and 1 Peter 1:22-25). Not every word in the Bible is written *to* us, obviously, but every word was written and preserved *for* us. But if we don't read it, prayerfully seeking to learn from it, how can we know God's principles for life? How can we be reminded of what Jesus said and taught?

The third gift is teachers (Ephesians 4:11-14). The Apostle Paul is clear that by placing ourselves where we can be taught by God-gifted teachers, we are built up to minister as we should; we will grow in Christ's likeness; and, we will not be tossed by waves and blown around on every wind. Do you make time to fellowship with believers who serve as mentors and teachers – especially those Christians in healthcare who have faced similar storms as yours and have learned how to navigate them in godly ways? If not, what's your excuse…you like being tempest-tossed and all wet?

With these three gifts in mind, let's look back on the storm accounts of Mark and Matthew. If the boys had been in-dwelled by the Holy Spirit, recalled God's Word and spent just a little time teaching each other rather than panicking, they wouldn't have asked, *"Who is this? Even the wind and the sea obey Him!"* For Scripture says of God,

> *Then they cried out to the LORD in their trouble, and He brought them out of their distress. He stilled the storm to a murmur, and the waves of the sea were hushed. They rejoiced when the waves grew quiet. Then He guided them to the harbor they longed for.*
>
> Psalm 107:28-30 (also see Psalm 65:7 and 89:8-9)

∽ The Sword in *Your* Mouth

Take the helmet of salvation, and the sword of the Spirit, which is God's word.

Pray at all times in the Spirit with every prayer and request, and stay alert in this with all perseverance and intercession for all the saints. Pray also for me, that the message may be given to me when I open my mouth to make known with boldness the mystery of the gospel. For this I am an ambassador in chains. Pray that I might be bold enough in Him to speak as I should.

Ephesians 6:17-20

Part of my definition of Christian healthcare is "exuding the love, wisdom, and power of the Holy Spirit." In this well-known passage by the Apostle Paul, we get a glimpse of what this means lived out in our practice.

- We are to engage the physical and spiritual world as soldiers for Christ. Our weapon for combatting evil and brokenness is the Holy Spirit, helping us wield God's powerful Word to advance His kingdom.

- In the Garden of Gethsemane, the disciples didn't yet have the Holy Spirit, so they failed to stay alert and intercede in prayer. We do have Him though. He helps us be alert for opportunities, have a heart to intercede appropriately, and persist in prayer as a standard of our practice.

- The Holy Spirit, if we desire and ask Him to, will give us the words to speak at the right time and in the right way (John 14:26; Luke 21:12-15).

- You can't use the excuse that you are bound by the system to keep your mouth shut. Paul considered himself every bit as much an ambassador and soldier in chains as out of them. He relied on the Holy Spirit to help him accomplish his assignment.

- Knowing that God Himself, the Holy Spirit, indwells you and is given to you as comforter and counselor ought to make you bold! Not arrogant but confident that the One who has authority in heaven and on earth, and who has called you to be witness to Him – telling of the things he has done for you and the loving mercy He has had on you – gifted you with the Spirit instructing your spirit to how to speak.

Daily the Holy Spirit desires to speak through you. Will you let Him?

IMAGE & LIKENESS

So long as people are being born,

God's image is constantly being created afresh.

So long as people continue to be born again,

God's likeness is increasingly revealed to the world.

⌒ God's Image & Likeness in Patients

Understanding humans are created in God's image and likeness (Genesis 1:26-27) can and should impact how we view and care for our patients. This truth imbues the recipients of our care with value and it gives our care the goals of moving or restoring individuals to their greatest capacity to fulfill God's intention for their lives as His image and likeness.

What does it mean to be created in God's image?

Humans all reflect (image) God's character and nature, though certainly to a lesser degree. For example, God is a living and eternal being; God has put eternity in our hearts and, barring a derangement, people want to, *and were intended to*, live now and into eternity. For a human being to live fully in the image of God requires them to also manifest the persons of the Godhead: Father, Son and Holy Spirit. With careful observation we can see how that comes to be. The Father, who wills and directs, so to speak, is imaged in the soul (emotions, intellect, memories, and will) of a person. The human body reflects the Son, for He alone became fully human, suffered the fatigues of humanity, and sweat drops of blood as it were in praying He wouldn't have to suffer and die. The Holy Spirit is best seen reflected in the born-again spirit of anyone who believes God and trusts the person and work of Jesus. Thus, Father, Son and Holy Spirit are imaged in our soul, body and capacity to have our spirit animated by grace through faith.

What does it mean to be created in God's likeness?

Humans are also made into God's likeness as they grow more like Him in His manifestations of integrity, morality, love and stewardship over creation. Humans were intended to conduct themselves as God would. When humanity fell in Eden, we observe that the damage, the marring, most adversely impacted humanity's likeness to God. This makes sense since holy God could no longer walk with unholy humanity, discipling and modeling His goodness.

So when we serve a patient and/or their friends or family, we are dealing with valuable creations made in God's image and likeness. In a Christian holistic view of the people, we minister to the Father as we teach the soul; the Son Jesus as we heal the body; and, the Holy Spirit as we speak to someone's spirit. Our goal ought to be to do whatever we can to help each aspect of the whole being fulfill to the greatest extent possible God's intention for her or him to be like Him – which one day all believers will fully be (1 John 3:2; also Matthew 22:37-40, 25:40).

ও Isaiah's Prophetic Calling for Us

When the advent season unfolds, almost all of us will at some point reflect on Isaiah's remarkable prophesy of our Messiah coming not once, but twice. Isaiah 9:1-7 opens with a brief promise foretelling of the child to be given to us at the first Christmas. The center of the passage tells what the Messiah will be called by His Father and followers after His resurrection and ascension. The prophecy closes describing our Messiah's rule and reign after He returns – in a sense, the Christmas yet to come.

As Christians who serve through healthcare, we ought to take a keen interest in this wonderful passage. Since we know we are created in Christ to become increasingly conformed to His image and likeness, the lofty and tumultuous Isaiah 9:2-5 ought to stir and thrill our hearts, for in it we get a glimpse of the cosmic intersection of our Christian faith and our healthcare vocation.

- From Isaiah 9:2: As the Divinely ordained star led the Magi from the East and the glory of the heavenly host blazed over the shepherds in their fields, we also shine God's Light into the darkness surrounding our patients today (Philippians 2:13-15).

- From Isaiah 9:3: As we beam light into dark places by telling others about the Light of the World, we help enlarge the kingdom of God, increase joy, and multiply rejoicing among the nations (Genesis 1:28).

- From Isaiah 9:4-5: As we use our privileged platform as Christians providing excellent healthcare – healing bodies, teaching souls and speaking to spirits – we stand beside our Savior in shattering oppressive yokes of

42

bondage and subduing the evil, wild things which oppose God and His best intentions for our patients (Ephesians 6:10-20).

As you hear music and messages commemorating the coming of Immanuel – God with us – celebrate that God's gift to humanity in Jesus has been given to you to share. May you receive from the same Holy Spirit who overshadowed Mary, raised Jesus from the dead and indwells you, everything you need to be generous in sharing your Savior in the Christmas season.

൧ Image, Likeness, & Reasoning

Then God said, 'Let Us make man in Our image, according to Our likeness.'... So God created man in His own image; He created him in the image of God; He created them male and female.

Genesis 1:26a, 27

"Come, let us discuss this/reason together," says the Lord.

Isaiah 1:18a, HCSB/NIV

In the beginning was the Word [Logos: thoughts, wisdom or logic revealed in words and/or deeds], *and the Word was with God, and the Word was God. He was with God in the beginning... The Word became flesh and took up residence among us.*

John 1:1-2, 14

Human beings are created in God's image and likeness. In part that means that unique among all created beings, people have the intended capacity to reason -- to consider information and then make a choice. To be human, (even if today we live as a fallen vestige of what we were and will one day be), is to be able to think, to debate with oneself, with others, and with God. We express considerations and conclusions in words of thought, writing, speech and prayer, and by our actions. This has many applications for us as citizens and as practitioners of healthcare.

Reasoning as Citizens

Sometimes a government pursues reporters and suppresses investigation and discourse in the press because journalists gather facts, ordering and reasoning through them in order to share unpleasant conclusions in words. Other times governments delay or deny equal treatment under the law for select groups who individually or collectively seek facts, reason through them and write, speak or pray publicly regarding their conclusions. When governments do these things, it may not only be political callousness or an abuse of justice. At its deepest level, it is an attack on God's image and likeness in individual and corporate humanity. Our nation's founding fathers and the framers of our Constitution and Bill of Rights understood this. That's why they codified the First and Second Amendments in the Bill of Rights.

Reasoning as Healthcare Professionals

The right of a healthcare practitioner to speak and act is under attack. Thinking can't be taken away, but words and actions can be assailed, stifling the ability to express reasoned conclusions, either in our words or deeds. Assaults on a healthcare worker's right of conscience is not just a danger to our livelihood. It goes to the heart of what it means for us and those we care for to be a human being in God's image and likeness. This

> To be human is to be able to think, to debate with oneself, with others, and with God.

is a grave matter. Right of conscience must be protected.

Two Applications of Reasoning & Image in Practice

A doctor friend of mine asked me two questions directly related to my point on reasoning in healthcare. I want to share them with you.

1. Our Non-Compliant Patients

Should we get mad, be frustrated, think less of, or write off patients who don't follow our instructions? Do we succumb to a temptation to be curt or ambivalent if our patients make choices other than what we recommend?

Certainly not. They are God's image and likeness just as we are. God calls us to reason and try persuasion based on our resources, skills, and experience, similar to how He used prophets like Ezekiel (see Ezekiel 3:1-21 and 33:1-20). We must allow that if, after a reasoned recommendation, a patient chooses an alternative course, you are seeing a manifestation of God through that person made in His image and likeness. Ours is not to suppress humanity or be angry because God created people to make choices.

2. Reasoning Through Guilt Over Poor Outcomes

The second question was about our regret or feeling guilty about mistakes. Should we detest the time we reflect on things we did in our patient care which seemed to go wrong? Is this effort counter-productive and a waste of time?

No. This inner conversation is a gift from God. It is a sign you are truly human. You reason through your actions, using words, so that you may reach a conclusion on whether you really made a mistake. If you did, learn from it and don't repeat it. Your mistakes prove you are not God. However, they can remind you that you bear His image and likeness.

May you begin to see yourself, your patients, your profession and your citizenship in a fresh way. God fashioned all of us in His image and likeness, with the ability to consider words, reason, and make and express choices – a precious human characteristic we need to cherish and protect.

∽ Why Linger in Dying?

"Why does my loved one (or, Why do I) linger in dying?" That's a tough question. Patients and loved ones ask it. Healthcare students are asking it. Many of you in practice or retirement have faced or asked such a question. I myself continue to engage with it. My wife Sandy went to heaven after months of withering away. My mentor Bill, also spent the better part of a year sitting in a wheel chair waiting for his failing heart to give out. Daily I would go to the 'rehabilitation center' to read Scripture to my brother in Christ, Elree, while his brain tumor grew and his tent slowly folded up. We all ask, in some way, "If the end is inevitable, why linger…why not just flip a switch and be done?" (I am being metaphorical here, *not* advocating euthanasia.)

The Theological and Hopeful Answer: Because of God's Image in People

When I was first forced to confront this question up close, a hospice nurse who was trying to be helpful would vacillate between saying it was the patient who had some mental issue they were wrestling with and so they were not 'ready to go,' or saying that a loved one had a 'mental or emotional reservation' and so wouldn't give the patient permission to go. In effect, the patient had to linger until one or both parties 'got their head straight.' I won't belabor the point of not only how painful this sort of 'help' is, but also how easily a few minutes of thought or reflection on the empirical evidence all around us refutes this exaggerated idea that people can

> Death is the
> last intimate thing
> we ever do.
> Laurell K. Hamilton

47

just will themselves or others to drop dead or hope themselves or others to never die. Empirical evidence and Christian theology both point us in an alternative direction to find our answer for why patients linger in their dying.

Empirical Evidence

First, the protective and redundant construction of the body, homeostasis, its immune system, and its recuperative powers all give evidence that the human body is organized to endure. In fact, according to the historical record, our antediluvian ancestors lived on the order of a millennium, and even today it is common to live a century, rather than days or weeks like a fly or potted plant. In general, it takes tremendous force or a cascade of failures to cause our body to die. Second, evidence also comes from our observations that we don't find dozens of dead bodies lying around our city streets every morning – even in terrible times of economic downturn, despair and hopelessness. People simply can't will their bodies to stop functioning when they don't want to live any more. (Try willing yourself to stop breathing.)

Christian Theology Explains the Evidence and Answers the Question

Humans are created in God's image, reflecting His character and nature. Part of God's nature is to be alive and live for eternity. Our bodies were intended to walk with God into eternity from the time they were fashioned and knit together in a fearful and wonderful way in our mother's womb. It is an afterglow of God's image in fallen humanity that God intended for us to physically endure in fellowship with Him, and so our bodies resist death with every means at their disposal. Death is counter to God's image.

Then why, you may ask, did God impose death upon humanity when Adam and Eve ate the fruit of knowledge of good and evil? Because without death, humanity would be destined to live forever in rebellion, growing less and less like God (and more and more like Satan). Death actually is a severe mercy. It offers those who accept God's call to reconciliation through Jesus a reset – an opportunity to walk with God as Adam and Eve once did.

Application

The next time a patient or a family member asks you why it takes some time for the body to give up the struggle to live, think about the theology of being created in God's image and likeness. Use their questions to point to God's love and plan for all people to be reconciled to Him and fellowship with Him forever as He first intended. Use this question as a springboard for offering the hope of the resurrection of the redeemed. Make this one of those special Romans 8:28-30 conversations, emphasizing that even at this late and difficult hour (like that of the thief on the cross), whoever calls on the name of the Lord will be saved…to live forever as a united body, soul and spirit!

❧ Help from the Garden

As the autumn leaves change and start to fall, the contemplative person recognizes that even though there are seasons that lead to browning, dying, and dropping, in this there is still purpose and beauty. There is also great hope and expectation for the future.

I mention this because the nagging search for answers to life's toughest situations, whether our own or those of our patients, are perennial. No matter where we are on the spectrum of practice, from student to retiring, we are asked to give hope and meaning to sometimes very stark or dark situations. Because we know the love of One who suffered, died and rose again for us, and we want to serve Him, it is natural that we want to be able to give His help and hope to those we encounter. But how? What can we say in times of turmoil and tribulation that doesn't come across as 'preachy?'

Two missionaries, I. Lilias Trotter and Elisabeth Elliot, recognized God's hand and plan in ordaining a season such as autumn. Seeing His hand behind what seems to be a portent of death and chill, these women wrote some of the most helpful literature the Christian community has on finding meaning in death and life. They use the testimony of the life cycle of seedbearing plants and trees to help us understand our own lives, the lives of those around us, as well as suffering and resurrection. This of course is most perfectly exemplified in the life of our Savior, Jesus Christ.

If you have been looking for ways to explain stages of life and death and new, resurrected life to those who ask you, may I suggest you take time to read one or more of these books? They are solidly Christian in theology and yet very accessible in relating the things we see in the flora around us to the challenges we face alongside our patients, families and friends. If you can only pick one book, I recommend choosing the more comprehensive and contemporary one: Elisabeth Elliot's *A Path Through Suffering: Discovering the Relationship Between God's Mercy and Our Pain*. The two much older and shorter books from Ms. Trotter are *Parables of the Christ-Life* and *Parables of the Cross*.

Priorities

Christian healthcare implies, in part,

practitioners have surrendered priority-setting to Jesus.

Satan, through the systems of this world,

would reset God's priorities.

Beware his schemes.

❧ Don't Confuse Calling with Vocation

When my wife Judy was headed to Athens and Thessaloniki, we read Acts 17 and 1 & 2 Thessalonians in preparation. I was struck by a passage addressing, in principle, a common confusion among Christians in healthcare. "Am I someone called to be a Christian who practices healthcare, or am I called to healthcare and happen to also be a Christian?" May I share some thoughts about this question with you?

There will come a day,

> *when He* [our Lord Jesus] *comes to be glorified by His saints and to be admired by all those who have believed, because our testimony among you was believed. And in view of this, we always pray for you that our God will consider you worthy of His calling, and will, by His power, fulfill every desire for goodness and the work of faith, so that the name of our Lord Jesus will be glorified by you and you by Him, according to the grace of our God and the Lord Jesus Christ.*
>
> 2 Thessalonians 1:9-12

First, it certainly appears that when Jesus returns, He won't be taking a census of our vocations. His concern will be whether we who believed the testimony we heard about Him, and thus were declared by God to be holy ones (saints), glorify and admire Him. When Jesus returns for us, our earthly jobs in healthcare (which do serve to ameliorate the effects of the fall) will perish with the fallen heavens and earth. However, praising God will go on forever in the new heavens and earth. That helps us to think about priorities from God's perspective.

Second, it is hearing and responding to God's calling us to follow Christ that instills in us the Holy Spirit empowered desire to do good and do our work by faith. That 'doing good' and 'work of faith' isn't obeying rules or acts of legalism. Nor is it our vocation *per se*. It is loving and serving our neighbors as ourselves (Galatians 5:6 & 13-14). In using our vocation, whatever it might be, as a vehicle for serving and loving our neighbors, we are living life in God's likeness, using the gifts, aptitudes and talents God has given us (1 Corinthians 4:7).

Finally, glorification certainly seems central to God's heart. It is not just that He receive all the glory and praise that is due to Himself. He wants to glorify those who responded in faithful believing to His calling them to Himself, too. He will use our vocation as a vehicle to bring us glory – if – we are using our vocation to bring glory to His name. To ensure that happens, out of the immeasurable abundance of His grace towards us, He enables us to testify about Him as part of our vocation.

Christian healthcare starts with the understanding we are called to follow Christ first. Our healthcare vocation is but one, temporary, aspect of how we do that.

❧ Finding Meaning in Finding Meaning

In "Surprised by Meaning" (*Kitchen Table Wisdom: Stories That Heal*, New York, Riverhead Books, 1996, pp. 159-162), Rachel Naomi Remen, MD relates an account of an ER doctor delivering a baby. Though he had delivered hundreds of babies, this delivery was different. As he suctioned the infant's nose, she opened her tiny eyes for the first time, looking the doctor right in his eyes. For the first time, he paused to gaze back. He realized that he was the first thing this little child ever saw. Such a thought pierced him. It gave what he had already done so many times before a new meaning. This child wasn't merely the object of professional competence or skilled procedures. This was a new human being launching out on a new life.

When our healthcare career is built on self-dependence, on trusting in our experience, competence, skills, etc., we gradually move into the realm of being a technician. Technicians get bored. They get burned out. They can, as I have seen and heard on many occasions, become disenchanted with their work because their technical prowess often provides only a temporary, and sometimes messy or painful, extension of the mortal life. "What's the point?" they ask.

> As Christians, our redeemed lives have meaning and purpose.

As Christians, our redeemed lives have meaning and purpose. It is a greater purpose to love and serve God by loving and serving our patients in His Name: to be His ambassadors, sharing His love and hope. It is to salt and light our encounters with the hope of eternal life through Christ, who through His resurrection has proven God desires to give victory to whosoever will over sin, broken bodies and minds, and over death.

Discover God's meaning for your life as a Christian minister serving humanity through healthcare. Let it empower you to see your patients with spiritual vision and to speak to them with a spiritual voice. Then you can walk through this world as Jesus did, letting your 'technical prowess' to heal bodies and teach souls serve as the opening to help your patients be spiritually born again, or find renewed hope in Jesus. Then they too can begin a whole new – eternal – life. And you will find enduring meaning in your work.

ॐ Simple Isn't Silly

My physician gave me a very simple instruction: Get exercise. Seeing the poor physical and mental results I achieved by not doing it, I followed his instructions. Voila! My weight dropped. My HDL went up. My A1C dropped. My mood went way up. When I obeyed his simple instruction my mess turned around.

The prophet Haggai was a man of simple instructions, too, managing to get five prophetic messages into only 38 verses. Embedded in his book is this statement from God:

> The LORD of Hosts says this: "Think carefully about your ways. Go up into the hills, bring down lumber, and build the [My] house. Then I will be pleased with it and be glorified," says the LORD. "You expected much, but then it amounted to little. When you brought the harvest to your house, I ruined it. Why?" This is the declaration of the LORD of Hosts. "Because My house still lies in ruins, while each of you is busy with his own house."
>
> Haggai 1:7-9

The LORD of Hosts doesn't begrudge anyone acquiring food, wine, clothing, shelter, etc. Nor is He against having a nice career or home (see Matthew 6:25-32). What He does object to, and will use circumstances to reverse, is putting ourselves and our priorities ahead of bringing Him glory through our obedience (see Matthew 6:26-33-34 and the balance of Haggai).

Simple Instruction 1

"Think carefully about your ways." Has your highest priority become the building of your own estate? Remember, Jesus

warned in the parable of the sower (Mark 4:18-19) that such thinking leads to choking fruitlessness. Not sure if your circumstances have become your priority? Honestly judge whether you are bearing spiritual fruit for the Master. To put it another way, what is the Lord's return on investment for the talents He has invested with you as a Christian ministering through healthcare? (Matthew 25:14-30; Acts 1:8)

Simple Instruction 2

"Go up into the hills, bring down lumber, and build the [My] *house."* It is not enough to recognize your situation and then wish things were different or that you were more fruitful. You have to DO SOMETHING. "Faith without deeds…." This command through Haggai was given to a people, not a person in particular. It is a shared effort where everyone participates. So don't be daunted. Rather, join with fellow believers in your Christian healthcare community to get training and the tools to be lifelong kingdom builders through your Christian healthcare calling.

On the surface, Haggai's words seem simple. As good academics know though, the best writing is succinct and intelligible; it is memorable and communicates for lasting change. So let's not confuse simple with silly. God is calling us to be thoughtful and fruitful for Him, bringing Him glory and gratitude in all things we do, including our practice of healthcare.

⫷ Thrown Down

Mark 13:1-2 opens the chapter with Jesus beginning a discourse on the signs of the end of the age of the Gentiles, the Great Tribulation, and the return of Jesus to establish His kingdom here on earth. While the specific temple marked out to have every stone "thrown down" was the temple at Jerusalem (the prophesy being fulfilled in 70 A.D. by Emperor Tiberius' Roman army), there is a principle at play that is applicable today. It has to do with where you work.

When Jesus spoke about the temple at Jerusalem, its construction had already been underway some 43 years. It was a monument to man's architectural ingenuity, engineering and technological prowess, and the devotion to the worship ministry that took place there. Israel had come a long way through a series of worship edifices: Moses' mobile tabernacle, Solomon's temple (destroyed by Nebuchadnezzar), Zerubbabel's temple (post-exile, which elicited simultaneous laughter and weeping), and now possibly the most magnificent edifice of all, Herod's temple.

> Today, one might argue, our healthcare symbol is the 10-15 story high cantilever crane.

In medicine, we find parallels. If you think about it, you can see them for yourself. The most obvious one though is the current massive consolidation in healthcare, which has been occurring over several years. Huge, very imposing complexes are filled with medical priests and priestesses and their gargantuan support staffs. One used to look at the staff of Asclepius as the symbol of medicine. Today, one might argue, our healthcare symbol is the 10-15 story high cantilever crane.

The cautionary questions are these: As disciples of Jesus, who practice the ministry of medicine, are you enamored by the trappings and resources at your disposal – the place you practice – or are you enamored with Jesus and His plans for your practice? Are you more focused on keeping the medical temple intact, or on being His temple, filled with His Holy Spirit empowering your medical ministry?

One day, every man-made structure and system will be thrown down, or more literally, violently shaken and then burned up. The King of kings will create a new heaven and a new earth. There will be no suffering or sickness. QED, there will be no need for medical temples or priests. Thus, the only enduring value in what you do each day is shepherding your patients, as appropriate, toward eternal life through Jesus. That activity is the only one taking place under the shadow of the cranes that won't be thrown down.

ᐒ   Not Willing that Any Should Perish

Sometimes we get so wrapped up in our expectations and traditional paradigms that we lose sight of immediate application of eternal concepts. So here is a challenge for you to take your expectations and paradigms to a new place in your practice. It is a way of speaking truth and life to patients who seem to have let themselves deteriorate physically or mentally, often because of guilt, unforgiveness, or a sense of hopelessness.

> *Dear friends, don't let this one thing escape you: With the Lord one day is like a thousand years, and a thousand years like one day. The Lord does not delay His promise, as some understand delay, but is patient with you, not wanting any to perish but all to come to repentance.*
>
> 2 Peter 3:8-9

God stands outside time but He understands that we are constrained by it. Often bad habits and self-destructive behavior take time to develop. They also take time to reverse. That's why Peter emphasizes God's patience in seeing us move in His direction. As we strive to live like Him (in His likeness), we not only have to have patience, but allow and encourage our patients to be patient with themselves, too. Change for the better takes time.

God also doesn't want *anyone* to perish. That means 'die responsible for their sins,' you say. True enough. But don't forget several other truths: God created this world as a place to promote the flourishing of each person's full potential. God has a plan for each person and has fearfully and wonderfully created them to fulfill that plan. Allowing the intended temple of the Holy Spirit to disintegrate due to self-abuse or neglect is a form of perishing.

Coming to repentance means coming to agree that God's ways, not ours, are the correct thoughts and behaviors. That includes having God's thoughts on the value and purpose of our bodies...you know, the very things Christ will return for at the rapture so He can call them out of the graves in an immortal, incorruptible, glorified state to be reunited with our soul and spirit and united with Him.

> God created this world as a place to promote the flourishing of each person's full potential.

So as healthcare practitioners walking in Jesus' footsteps, let's not forget to teach the emotions, intellect, memories, and will of our patients. God loves them and is patient with them. He wants to forgive them and give them hope. He asks them to think about themselves according to His good and gracious plans for them. He (and you) will patiently walk with them through the thinking and lifestyle changes that will save them from perishing.

~ Prepared for a Divine Encounter?

On the one hand, I am always encouraged to hear from Christians in healthcare about how they want to serve God in their studies or vocation. On the other hand, I am equally surprised at how unprepared we are to make the most of every divine encounter God gives us with our patients or peers. So without any need for editorial 'enhancement' I commend the following passage to you for personal meditation and reflection. Here you will find the keys to being prepared to serve God through your healthcare calling, even as you serve the whole person before you...body, soul, and spirit.

> *Devote yourselves to prayer; stay alert in it with thanksgiving. At the same time, pray also for us that God may open a door to us for the message, to speak the mystery of the Messiah, for which I am in prison, so that I may reveal it as I am required to speak. Act wisely toward outsiders, making the most of the time. Your speech should always be gracious, seasoned with salt, so that you may know how you should answer each person.*
>
> Colossians 4:2-6

⌒ Sought & Found

I was sought by those who did not ask;
I was found by those who did not seek Me.
I said: Here I am, here I am,
To a nation that was not called by My name.

Isaiah 65:1

The question this passage compels us to ask is, "How did God say to people not looking for Him, "Here I am?""

The Apostle Paul tells us,

But how can they call on Him they have not believed in? And how can they believe without hearing about Him? And how can they hear without a preacher? And how can't they preach unless they are sent? As it is written: "How beautiful are the feet of those who announce the Gospel of good things!"

Romans 10:14-15

You have a very privileged position as a Christian in healthcare. People come to you for care and advice. Certainly you have prepared to heal their bodies or teach their souls. However, do you also prepare yourself to speak to their spirit? By being deliberate about preparing and then appropriately exposing your patients to the loving person and work of Jesus, you are serving as God's ambassador, saying, "Here I am. Here I am."

May this be the year when you see the greatest fruitfulness in leading those who were not seeking God to find Him. May the Holy Spirit give you boldness to fully live your Christian life in your vocation of healthcare.

◌ Leaves, Your Tongue, & Healing

When God put mankind in the Garden of Eden, in its midst were the Tree of Life and the Tree of Knowledge of Good and Evil. God told Adam that if he ate from the latter tree then the curse of death would fall upon him. As our federal head, that curse fell upon all humanity when Adam didn't listen to God's Word but ate from the tree. The immediate result and cause of the promised death was being banished from access to the Tree of Life. [Interestingly, in his shame, Adam tried to cover Eve and himself with fig leaves. Imagine what eventually happens to our fig leaves when they dry up with time – they turn brown and crumble away.]

When God creates a new heaven and a new earth, in the midst of the New Jerusalem the Tree of Life reappears. *The tree of life was on both sides of the river [of living water], bearing 12 kinds of fruit, producing its fruit every month. The leaves of the tree are for healing the nations, and there will no longer be any curse"* (Revelation 22:2b).

Between our distant past and our future, King Solomon made an observation about a tree of life among us now. *The tongue that heals is a tree of life...* (Proverbs 15:4a). So we can say that our tongue exists to serve the same sort of healing role as the leaves of the tree of life. Our tongue can serve to set people free from the curse which befell humanity at Adam's fall. (By the way, have you thought about how similar in size and shape the visible portion of our tongue is to many kinds of tree leaves?)

The question then becomes, "How does a tongue bring healing from the curse of sin and death?" Simply put, the only cure for the curse of sin and death is Jesus Christ: *Christ has redeemed us from the curse of the law by becoming a curse for us, because it is written: "Everyone who is hung on a tree is cursed"*

(Galatians 3:13). The saving faith to trust in the person and work of Jesus Christ only comes one way – by hearing the Word of God.

> *But how can they call on Him they have not be-*
> *lieved in? And how can they believe without hear-*
> *ing about Him? And how can they hear without a*
> *preacher? And how can they preach unless they*
> *are sent? As it is written: 'How beautiful are the*
> *feet of those who announce the gospel of good*
> *things!'…So faith comes from what is heard, and*
> *what is heard comes through the message about*
> *Christ.*
>
> Romans 10:14-15, 17

You have many tools at your disposal for healing the body and/or teaching the soul of your patient. But do you use your special gift, your tongue, as a stand-in for a leaf from the tree of life, to heal spiritually? Do you speak to your patients as a contemporary tree of life, potentially setting them free from the curse of sin and death by exposing them to eternal life through Jesus Christ? A fig leaf won't save or heal. But the timely, appropriate words of your tongue, as a leaf from the tree of life, can.

[Editorial Note: Since the original writing of this Note of Encouragement, medical marijuana has become commonplace. Don't confuse my advocating for you to act as a leaf from the tree of life to heal with the rage to name pot dispensaries, The Healing Leaf. How quickly culture changes!]

❧ Christmas Angels Can Teach Much

The 1st Christmas Angel (Luke 1:5-20)

Gabriel appeared to the well-aged priest Zechariah while he served inside the temple. The religious man failed to recall God's work in the past and so was headed toward being a non-compliant doubter. Gabriel the messenger was able to transition from being a good news bearer to one who could confront the non-compliance in the authority he had been given. He could be stern, when the need arose.

The 2nd Christmas Angel (Luke 1:26-38)

Gabriel returns some months later to bring God's message of blessing to Mary. Mary exhibited complete trust in God and did not doubt what Gabriel was saying was true. She was, however, curious about how the message would come about…in a sense seeking details so she could give *informed* consent. Gabriel patiently took the time to explain the details to Mary's satisfaction. We all know how that worked out.

The 3rd Christmas Angel (Matthew 1:18-25)

An unnamed angel came to the betrothed Joseph in a dream. Joe was in a panic. His world was caving in. He was fearful of future events. The angel gave Joe context, purpose, and a reason to see this strange challenge through.

The 4th Christmas Angel and the Escorting Angelic Host (Luke 2:8-20)

Here the unnamed angelic army bursts into the mundane, day-to-day routine of shepherding life with glad tidings that have rung throughout the ages. Notice most importantly how God got the glory for giving the good news.

Angels aren't exactly subtle and I certainly haven't been too subtle, either. Angels are messengers, as are you. They served mankind, as do you. The angels tailored the way they presented their messages to the questions and responses of the person in front of them, as you do, too. The angelic messages were from God, as yours can be as well, when you share what the Lord has done for you and the loving mercy He has had on you.

May you see your role and responsibility as a messenger in a whole new light. Your name may remain anonymous, like that of so many of the angels, or it may be recorded for posterity like Gabriel's. In the end though, every one of the angels was chosen and sent by God to proclaim His message. You have been chosen as well. Take great heart in that wonderful news.

ᘖ Christmas Angels & You

You have probably noticed that when God wants us to know something is really, really important, He repeats Himself. Sometimes it is the Newer Testament writers quoting a passage from the Older Testament. Other times it is the sharing of accounts in the Gospels, or epistle writers hitting on the same messages. So when God sends an angel or two or three or an entire host (heavenly army) of them to key moments in the Christmas narrative, maybe we really ought to pay attention.

Why did God send angels over and over? Why were they so important? What application can we draw out by considering angels? What lesson do they have for us as Christians ministering to people through healthcare?

An Angel Is...

All of our English language translations of the Christmas accounts come from Greek manuscripts. There we find the Greek word *'angelos'*, which we transliterate 'angel.' Angel means 'messenger'...anyone who is a messenger, not only supernatural, ethereal beings.

You, good Christian sisters and brothers, are angels! It is in the very nature of our vocation and at the core of who Christians are called to be that we share God's messages of love, hope, forgiveness, and presence with our patients and peers.

❧ Springtime Frenzy & Priorities

Between taxes, conference invitations, the pull of spring cleaning, gardening and recreation opportunities, and our regular responsibilities, many of us are feeling a bit overwhelmed and overcommitted. We're trained to appear cool under pressure so we look like we have it all together and can accomplish the super human, but on the inside we might all be feeling a bit frenzied and somewhat guilty because we know we are going to have to turn down good things or break commitments we've already made.

So here are some brief thoughts on setting priorities, according to Biblical principles, which might help us feel less guilty and more successful in accomplishing the most important things in life. The central principle comes from Acts 1:8 and the promise that if you belong to Jesus you will be gifted with the indwelling Holy Spirit so that your whole life may be a supernaturally empowered witness to the things Jesus has done for you and the loving mercy He has had on you – in Jerusalem, Judea, Samaria, and the world.

> To find wisdom, I need to silence the demands of many to hear the commands of One.
>
> Glynnis Whitwer

Jerusalem

True and eternal success begins in Jerusalem, the place of the temple. *You are God's temple now.* Is God being worshiped and a daily, ongoing fellowship with Him happening in the temple? To condense important teachings of Jesus, 'If you love me, you will let me have lordship over every aspect of your being, even before loving your neighbors and one another' (John 14;15; Matthew 22:38-40; John

71

13:24-25). Any other definition of success is temporal, temporary, and likely aimed at feeding our cravings for human approbation or earthly security (review Matthew 6). Growth in God is the bulls-eye, the core. Don't miss the center for a peripheral.

Judea

The temple was surrounded by and embedded in Judea. We are (or ought to be) surrounded by and embedded in our family. They are the God-ordained first community. Their welfare and stewardship take precedence over everything else we are to care for (e.g., Deuteronomy 5:16, Malachi 2:13-16, Ephesians 5:22-6:4 or 1 Timothy 5:8). God doesn't command we entertain, indulge or spoil our families; we are to steward them unto godliness and flourishing. Are you hearing a siren's call away from accomplishing the latter? Be lashed to the cross, lest you and your family be dashed on the rocks.

Samaria

This was the place many Jews would pass through on their way to Judea and Jerusalem. Samaria does not represent our home. It is not a place to find an alternate temple to worship in. It represents the place of our vocations and our avocations. It is the place where God provides the resources to meet the needs of our families and ourselves. Here is where we mingle with the world on a regular basis, both performing work as ministry (since everything we do ought to be done as if unto the Lord) and loving our neighbors and one another. It is an important place, filled with Divine appointments, if you are looking for them. But it is not God's temple, nor is it the place of our primary stewardship responsibilities.

The World

Even in its broken state, the world is still a beautiful place, filled with a kaleidoscope of peoples whom God loves. We want to go on tours and trips for ministry and evangelism if we are able. However, if you are not faithful at letting the Lord supernaturally shape you in your Jerusalem, Judea, and Samaria, what exactly makes you believe you are going to be effective at great things on a global scale? It is those faithful to the 'little' things entrusted to them who will be given greater responsibilities. Again, don't miss the core for a peripheral.

Application

Do you want to be less stressed about having so much to do? Do you want to reduce the guilt over having to say 'No' to a request or offer, or over breaking a commitment? Then take heart in what Jesus has already freed you to do. Filter your scheduling through Biblical principles, like those of Acts 1:8. If you can honestly meet a request or desire without missing your essential central responsibilities, then joyfully "Let your 'Yes' be 'Yes.' " If you can't, then you have the Lord's permission to "Let your 'No' be 'No,' " without having to feel guilty about it.

May the Holy Spirit remind you of Jesus' teachings as you are confronted with your myriad of decisions and choices. May you know His peace as He helps you to make godly decisions and commitments, joyfully and free of guilt.

☙ Cry Out!

Suddenly there was a multitude of the heavenly host with the angel, praising God and saying: "Glory to God in the highest heaven, and peace on earth to people He favors!"

Luke 2:13-14

Now He [Jesus] came near the path down the Mount of Olives, and the whole crowd of the disciples began to praise God joyfully with a loud voice for all the miracles they had seen: "The King who comes in the name of the Lord is the blessed One. Peace in heaven and glory in the highest heaven!" Some of the Pharisees from the crowd told Him, "Teacher, rebuke Your disciples." He answered, "I tell you, if they were to keep silent, the stones would cry out!"

Luke 19:37-40

At both ends of Jesus' incarnational ministry, God's followers, be they angelic or human, were willing to come down from their heights to proclaim glory to God. Only those who thought highly of themselves or their man-made doctrines and commands insisted on silence rather than praise.

Jesus, however, would have nothing to do with silence when it came to giving God praise. All creation, no matter the form, owes its Creator God glory and praise. He will receive it one way or another.

Historically, those of us in healthcare have held lofty positions in our communities and have been held in high regard by our patients. I am so glad I have met so many wonderful Christian healthcare providers willing to declare the praises

74

of God through their patient care ministry. I hope in the coming year to meet even more of you and encourage you all to join with angels, people, and all creation in declaring the glory of God boldly!

⮎ Entrusted by Our Master

When we read about the apostle Paul, he, like so many of us, had the habit of describing his life as a collection of segments. Depending upon his circumstances, he referred to himself as a Hebrew, a Pharisee, a wicked man yet least of the apostles, a spiritual father, and a tentmaker. Once the Lord Jesus got ahold of him though, Paul's life consolidated around a unifying theme and purpose. This purpose was irrespective of the particular activity or vocation he might have been engaged in at any particular time. Paul described his purpose as follows –

> *Paul, a slave of God and an apostle of Jesus Christ, to build up the faith of God's elect and their knowledge of the truth that leads to godliness, in the hope of eternal life that God, who cannot lie, promised before time began. In His own time He has revealed His message in the proclamation that I was entrusted with by the command of God our Savior.*
>
> Titus 1:1-3

What is the unifying theme and purpose of your life? As a Christian practicing the vocation of healthcare, you too belong to Jesus Christ. You have been given the Gospel and commissioned to take it everywhere you go, in Christ's authority (Matthew 28:18-20). You've been declared Christ's ambassador – messenger (2 Corinthians 5:18-21). You are also Jesus' agent sent to comfort those who are afflicted (2 Corinthians 1:3-5).

We are all so busy and lead segmented lives, just as Paul did. However, let's not ever lose sight of the eternal purposes of God and how He has given His purpose to our lives, just as

76

He did for the Apostle Paul. No matter what you are spending your time doing, may the Holy Spirit remind you frequently of the ultimate purpose God has entrusted you with. May you be faithful in serving our Lord and Master Jesus by daily living out His purposes through you.

When you realize God's purpose for

your life isn't just about you,

He will use you in a mighty way.

Dr. Tony Evans

❧ Live by Faith

We strive through our healthcare practice to help people live to the healthiest and fullest extent possible and to minimize suffering. The rub sometimes comes in defining what living means, for the definition often slides from objective to subjective. As Christians performing the ministry of healthcare, we have God's Word to help us bring clarity to the meaning and goal of helping people abundantly live – now and forevermore. That sets us apart from all others in our profession. But do we avail ourselves of the resource? Does it guide our care?

In about 615 BC, God was describing to Habakkuk the state and pending judgment of the proud, the arrogant and merciless, etc., when He slipped in this 'tiny' statement: *But the righteous one will live by his faith* (Habakkuk 2:4). This wasn't a new idea. God had given a similar statement to Isaiah some 110 years prior when speaking of a similar situation: *If you do not stand firm in your faith, then you will not stand at all* (Isaiah 7:9b).

In the first century AD, the author of Hebrews and the Apostle Paul saw these small sentences have big ramifications and so incorporated life-by-faith into their teaching as foundation stones.

> *For yet in a very little while, the Coming One will come and not delay. But My righteous one will live by faith; and if he draws back, I have no pleasure in him. But we are not those who draw back and are destroyed, but those who have faith and obtain life.*
>
> Hebrews 10:37-39

78

Now it is clear that no one is justified before God by the law, because the righteous will live by faith.

Galatians 3:11

For I am not ashamed of the gospel, because it is God's power for salvation to everyone who believes, first to the Jew, and also to the Greek. For in it God's righteousness is revealed from faith to faith, just as it is written: The righteous will live by faith.

Romans 1:16-17

If we take our healthcare ministry seriously, and our goal is the best life possible for our patients, then we are confronted by these texts with two questions. Our patients must live by faith in what or whom? How might they come to that faith? The Apostle Paul answered both in one short statement.

But how can they call on Him they have not believed in? And how can they believe without hearing about Him? And how can they hear without a preacher? And how can they preach unless they are sent? As it is written: "How beautiful are the feet of those who announce the gospel of good things!"... So faith comes from what is heard, and what is heard comes through the message about Christ.

Romans 1:14-15, 17

You, sisters and brothers, are the Ambassadors with Beautiful Feet, bringing life (2 Corinthians 5:16-21). As you practice your healthcare ministry, remember it is your privileged position to *expose* (not impose) the life found by faith in Jesus as you heal the body and teach the soul of your patients. In doing so and speaking to your patient's spirit, you help bring real, abundant, eternal life.

79

❧ Thinking About Calling vs. Vocation

A Reflection on Psalm 90, Psalm 39, and Ephesians 2:10

This short life is not about what we *do* in this world but who we *are* in Him.

> This is our eternal calling.

However, what we do in this short life reveals Him – and, by extension, us in Him – to this world.

> This is our temporary vocation.

We are called to follow Christ first. Our healthcare vocation is but one, temporary, aspect of how we do that.

LOVE

The greatest of these is love.

Love never ends.

❧ Musings on Love in Healthcare

Did you ever wonder where the brilliant Apostle Paul might have come down on the subject of love? Being a man with a deep soul and able to move between the emotional and intellectual realms with superb grace, we shouldn't be surprised his writing on love is some of the world's most oft-quoted. After all, he declared love to be, "the most excellent way." If Paul thought so much of love, maybe now is a good time to reflect upon how it applies to our Christian healthcare practice.

Just as we depend a great deal upon context when listening to and diagnosing our patients, Paul was very much a student of context. That's why he might chafe somewhat if he were to see his great love poem 1 Corinthians 13 co-opted as a stand-alone sonnet on a greeting card. It is not that the words aren't true or can't stand by themselves, but they lose some of their most important meaning and power when taken out of context. (After all, a runny nose, without context, could simply be a cold. In context, it may actually indicate a seasonal allergy or be revealed as leaking CSF.)

So what was the context of Paul's love treatise? Paul spoke of the variety of gifts God gave, by the Holy Spirit, to build one another up in 1 Corinthians 12. In 1 Corinthians 14, Paul gave examples of practical and tangible ways those gifts are to be applied in community with one another. The point of 1 Corinthians 13 then can clearly be understood as it was intended. God gifts us to serve one another – by, with and in love – in practical and orderly ways, so that all of us are built up as God would have it.

As Christians involved in healthcare, we can draw great wisdom from the words and ideas of Paul. We find we have been gifted and put in community to serve community.

From 1 Corinthians 12, do we let the Holy Spirit empower our gifts, or do we strive daily to gin them up in our own strength? From 1 Corinthians 14, we see we should use our gifts in a fashion that reflects God to the watching world. Are we as thoughtful, circumspect and orderly as our God is? Finally, the great 1 Corinthians 13 reminds us that at the heart of it all – the most excellent way – is letting the love of God infuse our gifts and how we use them. Otherwise, calling ourselves providers of Christian healthcare turns out to have only a noisy, hollow ring to it.

May the Lord fill you with joy over His great love for you. May you discover an excellent way to share it with your loved ones, peers and patients.

ல Love through Christian Healthcare

Valentine's Day urges upon us thoughts of love. Whether it is our children in elementary school giving a valentine card to every student in class to demonstrate brotherly affection, or the sweet whisperings shared between a husband and wife in private, now is the season to express love.

How do you express love through your practice of medicine or dentistry? Is the love for your patients worldly? Is it indistinguishable from that of your peers who have not yet come to put their faith in Jesus? One might imagine that your love for your patients, at a minimum, ought to look at least as shiny as that of your unbelieving peers. However, the God who loves us so much He was willing to die for us, thinks our love as His followers ought to be far brighter and much more distinguishable. It should exceed that of other practitioners, because of the Person and power behind it. "How?" you ask.

> Kind words can be short and easy to speak, but their echoes are truly endless.
>
> Mother Teresa

Let's begin to answer that by envisioning some realities of our practice. In our rapidly transforming healthcare paradigm, we encounter some patients we would never count as friends, administrations asking the white coat off our back, and reimbursements that simply don't add up. But this is really nothing new. In Luke, Jesus taught His followers how to engage those who despise us, those who demand our labor, and those who don't want to pay us what is reasonably owed to us. Love them!

But it's not with any ol' love. It is God's love, manifest through us. Jesus said,

> *Love your enemies, do what is good to those who hate you, bless those who curse you, pray for those who mistreat you. ...If you love those who love you, what credit is that to you? Even sinners love those who love them. ...But love your enemies, do what is good, and lend, expecting nothing in return. Then your reward will be great, and you will be sons of the Most High. For He is gracious to the ungrateful and evil.*

> Luke 6:27-36

Love your patients, peers, and co-workers in Christian love. Honor your Heavenly Father by emulating His love. Challenging as that might occasionally be, your great reward might turn out to be setting someone on the path to eternal life through Christ Jesus.

↪ The Whosoever Wills

*For the scripture saith, Whosoever believeth on
him shall not be ashamed. For there is no difference
between the Jew and the Greek; for the same Lord
over all is rich unto all that call upon him. For
whosoever shall call upon the name of the Lord
shall be saved.*

Romans 10:11-13, KJV

Working in emergency medical services for years, I encountered and cared for people most of society drives by at intersections, locks their car doors against when driving through their neighborhoods, or steps around in parks and alleyways. These folks are the ones who, for a variety of reasons, have become part of "the poor you will always have with you." Sadly, being poor often is found in the company of substandard education, diet, shelter, hygiene, and healthcare for body and soul.

Sometimes even the caregivers don't want to be around people with so many problems. Weary of smells, behaviors, and chronically poor decision making, practitioners can become jaded, hardened, and even abusive towards these people. If I were practicing healthcare from a purely flesh-based standard, I might have fallen into the same mindset.

However, as a follower of Jesus Christ, I didn't practice fleshly healthcare. I used my privileged position to minister to the poor through Christian healthcare. The standard I tried to use for providing care was that of Jesus. It is found in Mark 12:28-34. In a nutshell, Jesus says that as we vertically love God with all we are, and we horizontally love our neighbors as we love ourselves, we are not far from the kingdom of God. One could say that as we practice healthcare in this way, we hold up the cross of Christ before a watching world.

I don't say that last bit in a purely metaphorical way. Time and time again, caring with the mind of Christ – a mind of sacrificial love, valuing all life, and desiring that none should perish – made the jaded pause. What was happening that someone could love the unlovely in such a way? Many times partners and fellow first responders would ask me weeks later how and why I could treat the despised with such uncommon care. My answer was generally the same. God loves and values everyone, and so as His follower I strive to as well. The love is the Holy Spirit's love working through me.

> The only question you have to ask yourself is whether you want to care for the whosoever wills as much as Jesus does.

You follow the same Savior and Lord. You are indwelled by the same Holy Spirit. Everything you need to live the cross of Christ through your healthcare practice is available to you. You too can love the unlovely. The only question you have to ask yourself is whether you want to care for the whosoever wills as much as Jesus does.

❧ And Your Excuse Is ...?

> *I appeal to you, instead, on the basis of love. I, Paul, as an elderly man and now also as a prisoner of Christ Jesus, appeal to you for my son, Onesimus. I fathered him while I was in chains.*
>
> Philemon 1:9-10

We are all very busy. We have issues. Busy plus issues all too often equals excuses.

Paul was busy too, evangelizing the Gentiles anywhere and everywhere he could get to them (see Acts 17:16-30, for example). And we are reminded from his letter to Philemon that Paul had issues as well: he was an elderly man and he was chained up in a Roman prison. Yet, none of this seemed to excuse him from loving others into the kingdom of God.

If we love God, and if we love people as God loves them and are troubled by their lostness, then that love should work itself out through us. It will not be overcome by excuses rooted in issues and busyness. Motivated by love, we will appeal to the wisdom and power of the Holy Spirit and God's Word to help us find a way to expose our peers and patients to the love of Jesus. God has a marvelous way of using our availability and His work to birth new children into His family. Don't you want to be a part of that?

Busy + issues

all too often

= excuses.

HOPE

Certainly, the life is in the blood.

Wisdom literature tells us, however,

the power to make the heart pump it is hope.

ᐧ The Hope You Have to Offer

"I hope I won't need a root canal."

"I hope this IV won't hurt."

"I hope he can get my disease under control."

"I hope this is the right medicine without bad side effects or dangerous interactions."

"I hope she can show me how to resolve my despair."

"I hope they can teach me to walk, talk, or brush my teeth again."

"I hope she can wake me up afterwards."

"I hope they save me."

We've all heard our patients or their family members make comments like this – sometimes with a smile or sometimes through tears. Day after day, hour after hour, person after person is looking to *you* to satisfy their hope. No pressure on you, eh?

Thank God daily that He has gifted and called you into the ministry of healthcare. It is a privileged responsibility. Thank Him as well that through His Word illuminated by the power of His Holy Spirit, we recognize we are to minister skillfully and joyfully (Psalm 33:3) but not be gods in charge of making life flourish (1 Corinthians 3:5-7).

Part of what makes your position so privileged is that not only might the Lord wonderfully use you to meet the temporal hopes of your patients, but He has placed you in a position to offer or bolster a spiritual hope. This is the hope which will last up until the moment of its fulfillment when

God raptures our broken bodies as new, immortal, incorruptible, and glorious. No more groaning of body or soul (1 Corinthians 15:50-58).

Are you prepared to speak God's hope into the lives of your patients, peers and partners who are seeking real, lasting hope? Do you make a point of testifying to the hope *you* have because of what the Lord has done for you and the loving mercy He's had on you? (Mark 5:18-20)

May I suggest that you find ten minutes sometime this week to (re)read Romans 5:1-11 and 8:18-28. Pray over these words and ask God to help you commit their principles to heart. Then, when your patient or their family looks to you for hope, you'll not only be ready to offer them whatever hope your skills and wisdom can, but even more so, be ready to offer them God's sure and enduring hope – a hope you can personally testify is your hope, too.

> *Now may the God of hope fill you with all joy and peace in believing, so that you may overflow with hope by the power of the Holy Spirit.*
>
> Romans 15:13

✍ You & the Tree of Life

Before God Almighty created Adam, (at the time the only human and thus our federal head), the LORD placed the Tree of Life at the heart of the Garden of Eden. Nearby was the Tree of the Knowledge of Good and Evil. God gave Adam free will and reason: attributes of His image. He allowed Adam to exercise these by giving him a choice. God said, "If you choose to eat from the latter tree, on that day you will certainly die."

Subsequently, Adam ate from that tree. Yet the Biblical record shows he didn't die that day – not in body, soul, or spirit. So if God wasn't wrong, or a liar, what did He mean? According to the account in Genesis 3:22-24, the Lord meant that humanity would be barred from access to the Tree of Life. Rather than having His creation remain in a perpetual state of unholy rebellion against Himself, God meted out the consequence of lost access to the Tree of Life, leading to eventual bodily death – a *severe mercy*. Apart from the *severe mercy of death*, (which is the wage of sin), there could be no redemption, declaration of imputed righteousness through Christ, or reconciliation with God.

> To keep this new body alive, the Tree of Life awaits us in heaven.

For those who are, by grace through faith in the person and work of Jesus, redeemed and reconciled to God, the bodily resurrection is the hope of their future. And behold! To keep this new body alive, the Tree of Life awaits us in heaven. Only through overcoming faith in Christ can anyone partake of its 12 fruits, monthly new crop, and leaves which are for the healing of the nations from the curse of sin (see Revelation 2:7, 22:1-3a, and 22:12-21).

The implication of this appears to be humans were not created immortal. Immortality was not lost at the Fall. Rather, God made provision for us that so long as we have access to the fruit and leaves of the Tree of Life, through obedience to God, we live on in health.

Solomon, using similes, foreshadowed that the Tree of Life has a part in Christian healthcare today.

- Proverbs 3:18 says God's wisdom is a tree of life – Christ is our wisdom.

- Proverbs 11:30 says righteousness is a tree of life – Christ is our righteousness.

- Proverbs 13:12 says we need fulfilled hope and desire – Christ is our hope and desire.

- Proverbs 15:4 says the way we speak is a tree of life – Jesus calls us to speak healing and loving truth.

If Jesus can say that He is the vine and we are the branches, and if the leaves on the Tree of Life are for the healing of the nations, then it is not a stretch to say that through our Christian healthcare, we are like leaves on the Tree of Life when we speak to those we encounter about where true wisdom, righteousness, and hope are found – in Christ Jesus. This is the pathway to eternal healing.

☙ Hopeful Prescriptions

Isaiah 40 is a remarkable chapter about sin and forgiveness, the crooked and straight, the difference between man's condition and God's eternal perfection, and our brokenness and God's offer of eternal healing. The thread woven between all these ideas is the role of the herald, which is where we as Christian healthcare practitioners come in.

We serve those who have broken lives: failing bodies, disturbed souls, or maybe they are still in a state of having a spirit yet unborn – dead to God. Some of our patients will think that God doesn't care about them or listen to them: they feel hopelessly in bondage to addiction, guilt, or shame. Some others will despair because their body is betraying them, even unto disability or death. Finally, others will have no hope for a future because they don't yet know the One in whom they can put their hope. In all of these situations, you as the herald might want to take them to the following two passages. They may be the prescriptions your patient really needs.

> *Jacob, why do you say, and Israel, why do you assert: "My way is hidden from the LORD, and my claim is ignored by my God"? Do you not know? Have you not heard? Yahweh is the everlasting God, the Creator of the whole earth. He never grows faint or weary; there is no limit to His understanding. He gives strength to the weary and strengthens the powerless. Youths may faint and grow weary, and young men stumble and fall, but those who trust in the LORD will renew their strength; they will soar on wings like eagles; they will run and not grow weary; they will walk and not faint.*
>
> Isaiah 40:27-31

Grace to you and peace from God our Father and the Lord Jesus Christ. Blessed be the God and Father of our Lord Jesus Christ, the Father of mercies and the God of all comfort. He comforts us in all our affliction, so that we may be able to comfort those who are in any kind of affliction, through the comfort we ourselves receive from God. For as the sufferings of Christ overflow to us, so our comfort overflows through Christ. ...And you can join in helping with prayer for us, so that thanks may be given by many on our behalf for the gift that came to us through the prayers of many.

2 Corinthians 1:2-5, 11

It wasn't God's original intent that the whole world would groan with afflictions, but sin has consequences. So now as descendants of the first Adam we all encounter pressures, trials, and maybe even terrors at one time or another. Whether in our practice or personal lives, each of us is old enough to recognize and relate to this truth.

However, we are Christians. That means we have made a commitment to put our faith for complete forgiveness and eternal life in Jesus Christ, the second Adam, who is making all things new in due season. While sin and humanity's fall still have consequences, they are no longer of eternal consequence to us AND, until we go home to heaven, we don't have to face afflictions alone.

> It wasn't God's original intent that the whole world would groan with afflictions, but sin has consequences.

The theologian in me would like to wax rhapsodic about this truth as it relates to this passage from 2 Corinthians. Instead, I'll just refer you also to Hebrews 2:14-18 and John 14.

95

Viewing these three passages together, you'll discover the remarkable concept that grace, peace, and mercy from our Heavenly Father in our times of affliction are incarnate in Christ. And the promised comfort? It too is not an action, *per se*, but the person of the indwelling Holy Spirit. Our Heavenly Father loves those who love His Son so much that He gave both His Son and His Holy Spirit to come alongside us in our afflictions, with all the authority, power and wisdom of the Godhead as our ever-present hope and help in times of trouble.

Application

The Apostle Paul made note at the end of this statement that his ability to clearly communicate this Gospel truth to those who needed comfort, as well as those who were under affliction, came as a result of praying saints. When you enter a classroom, an exam room, a surgical suite, or the presence of a suffering friend or family member, do you make a point of praying for and with those who are afflicted? You bear in yourself God, but do you share His comfort by introducing Him to the hurting? All of our various professional healthcare ministrations may bring temporary relief, which is good. But they don't bring the lasting comfort our *Abba* Father desires to give. Only His is a comfort that lasts eternally. And you, dearest friends, may well be Divinely appointed to be the agent of grace who brings that comfort to the afflicted. Will you?

May God be YOUR all-sufficient comforter. As you praise Him with gratitude in your heart and on your lips, may He use you to comfort others with the comfort He has given you. You are loved by God. Receive and share it.

ᕼ Healing Broken Spirits

When humans come to the end of themselves, when they have no hope for the future because they can find no way to alter their adverse circumstances, Scripture says they reach a place of crisis. They have a broken spirit. In Job 17:1, Job lamented what it was like to have a broken spirit: *My spirit is broken. My days are extinguished. A graveyard awaits me.* The writer of Proverbs 18:4 says that Job's experience potentially comes to all mankind at one point or another: *A man's spirit can endure sickness, but who can survive a broken spirit?* A broken spirit, according to this same writer, is damaging to both body and soul.

Yet there is a remedy for the broken spirit and the wounds it causes. According to Proverbs 15:13 and 17:22 respectively, the cure is a joyful heart. *A joyful heart makes a face cheerful, but a sad heart produces a broken spirit*, and *A joyful heart is good medicine, but a broken spirit dries up the bones.* The choice of the word 'joyful' is no accident. Happiness comes from being pleased with circumstances; joy exists outside our circumstances.

> The paradox of a joyful heart contra a broken spirit is that God delights in us having a broken spirit and heart!

A heart which can be at peace *regardless* of circumstances is one experiencing joy.

The paradox of a joyful heart contra a broken spirit is that God delights in us having a broken spirit and heart! *The sacrifice pleasing to God is a broken spirit. God, You will not despise a broken and humbled heart* (Psalm 51:17).

How can this be? Because when we reach that 'crisis point' of recognizing we have come to the end of ourselves – that place of humility and a broken spirit –we potentially become willing and able to turn things completely and fully over to God for His care and control. That includes trusting Him with our eternal destiny, which is unaffected by and outside our current circumstances. Only when we allow God to give us the hope found in trusting Jesus alone – hope which brings eternal joy – can we find true, enduring healing for everything which ails our soul and body.

As we minister in our healthcare settings, we will sometimes discern we are ministering to someone who has, or is near to having, a broken spirit. As Christians, we take seriously the Apostle James' admonition in James 2:16-17 against wishing someone well and then doing nothing to make provision for that.

What can we say or do for those of a broken spirit who need the joy of the Lord in their heart? One short, brief possibility is to point them to the words of Jesus, found in Luke. If you find comfort and joy in them, declare this as *your* story. Let the Holy Spirit and your patient then lead you where the conversation goes from there. No matter what happens, your well wishes will have been accompanied by the deed of offering the source of joy to the broken-spirited person.

> *Then looking up at His disciples, He said: "Blessed are you who are poor, because the kingdom of God is yours. Blessed are you who are hungry now, because you will be filled. Blessed are you who weep now, because you will laugh. Blessed are you when people hate you, when they exclude you, insult you, and slander your name as evil, because of the Son of Man. Rejoice in that day and leap for joy! Take note—your reward is great in heaven, because this is the way their ancestors used to treat the prophets."*

> Luke 6:20-23

May this be the year when you yourself prosper in body and soul, experiencing the joy of the Lord. As you do, may you be given the Holy Spirit empowered boldness to speak God's words of joy into the lives of those you touch, bringing good medicine to those with a broken spirit.

❧ Job Needed an Interventionist

Job's Situation

Having the benefit of biblical hindsight and, in particular, the Gospel, we know that blameless Job didn't need just information about the source of his boils, the sorrows of his soul, or his hopeless spirit. Job needed an interventionist who could minister healing to him on all three levels.

Job lacked the information that Satan existed and was hell-bent on destroying him in order to shame God. Without that information, Job thought God was persecuting him for no reason.

Job lacked the information that there is a future after death and that life doesn't end with Sheol – the place of the dead. Without hope for something greater in his relationship with God and for a dwelling place with Him, the acute and complete loss of the sense of mortal blessing led to Job's profound despair and his sinful behavior.

Much of what Job's friends said to him was correct information. But it didn't address the reality of Job's situation and was thus worse than unhelpful, leading to grief upon grief. Their counsel didn't point to the place where Job would find rest from his weariness and burden – the bosom of Christ (Matthew 11:28-30).

Job *did* know that he needed someone to stand between his fallibility and pain and God's holiness and omnipotence. Job *did* know that he needed an interventionist (Job 9:32-35). Job's friends didn't have any idea who that was – *worthless physicians, all of you* (Job 13:4). Job didn't know Him either – but he wanted to.

But I know my living Redeemer, and He will stand on the dust at last. Even after my skin has been destroyed, yet I will see God in my flesh. I will see Him myself; my eyes will look at Him, and not as a stranger. My heart longs within me.

Job 19:25-27

Application

People aren't coming to us just for information, though that is essential in order for them to make choices and give informed consent. More than information, people come to us for an intervention. Thankfully, most who come to us aren't in the state of calamity and collapse that Job was. However, as Christian healthcare providers, we ought to be the first to recognize that treating only one component of our patient, such as their body or soul, is an incomplete intervention. A complete intervention on our part is to speak truth to our patients about the one true interventionist – Jesus.

When the Holy Spirit prompts you that it is needed and appropriate, be bold enough to declare Satan is the enemy of our souls, tempts us to sin, and then accuses us of being unholy failures. He is the author of tempting lies and illness. Declare God loves us unconditionally and doesn't want to harm us, though He may test or discipline us to get our attention. Tell your patients the ultimate interventionist is Jesus Christ, whom you serve. He came to take our sins upon Himself so we might be found righteous in Him. The proof of God's power for ultimate healing is found in Jesus' resurrection from the dead to stand at the Father's right hand intervening for us now. Scripture promises one day He will stand again on this earth and those of us who have trusted Him will see our perfect, all-healing interventionist face to face (Isaiah 53:5, 12; 1 Corinthians 13:10-13).

May you see yourself as an interventionist who can speak God's truth into the lives of those around you, whether patient, peer, or partner. May you be the one whom God can count on to boldly go with the hurting to Jesus, our Great Interventionist.

GRATITUDE

Happiness rides upon

the black caterpillar of temporal circumstances.

Joy flies forever free as a polychromatic butterfly.

Gratitude is the cocoon of metamorphosis.

ぞ Thankful Thoughts from Prison

All of us really do have so much to be thankful for, because we have joy rooted in the timeless hope given by God. Thus our joy is eternal, unlike happiness, which is dependent upon temporal circumstances. To help us onto the path of thanksgiving, here's a brief thought.

Often referred to as the epistle of joy, the Book of Philippians is also an epistle of healing. Written from prison, the Apostle Paul speaks of how God heals our broken relationship with Him. He commends healing our minds by having the mind of Christ. The imprisoned apostle also urges healing among believers of damaged or broken relationships.

Paul offers a wonderful recommendation for staying healed. Rather than dwelling on brokenness and things which divide, Paul tells the church,

> Finally, brothers, whatever is true, whatever is honorable, whatever is just, whatever is pure, whatever is lovely, whatever is commendable – if there is any moral excellence and if there is any praise – dwell on these things. Do what you have learned and received and heard and seen in me, and the God of peace will be with you.
>
> Philippians 4:8-9

The one thing all of those adjectives might define is other people ... Paul using himself as an example. As we think about the best things in other people, God will be with us in peace. What a lovely thought! As Christians in healthcare, who make a vocation of engaging with so much that is broken, let's use thanksgiving to experience some healing and peace of our own. Let us enter into the presence of God by thinking about who has helped us, inspired us, discipled us, counseled us, or encouraged us by their words and deeds. Be an agent of grace and peace by telling them you thank God for all they have meant to you. Consider giving a card to your peers or staff with a simple one or two sentences about what worthy thing you see and appreciate in them. They will be blessed, you will be a blessing, and God will be glorified.

☙ Thankful for God's Love & Provision

After all the winter weather wackiness, isn't it wonderful to benefit from the blessings of springtime blooms and berries? Dogwoods, azaleas, rhodies, strawberries, etc. Our wonderful God has made these for our pleasure and to show His creative love to us. Let's be sure to thank Him, shall we?

At this time of year, schools and medical training programs are winding down, residents and fellows are coming and going, and practitioners are seemingly busier than ever. It is a time when transitions are the norm and everyone has more they would like to do than they have time for. So let us just encourage you that we are praying for you and wishing you God's very best. He loves you. Don't let vacation planning or work issues keep you from remembering and experiencing that.

↝ Every Day Is a Gift

The story is told of a church elder who had been called into an ICU room to pray for the healing of a person in his church who was at the threshold of the next world. This was an elder who took the admonition and instruction to pray for the sick seriously, including inviting the sick to confess any known sins (James 5:13-20).

After fulfilling his ministry to the patient, the elder did something curious. Looking squarely into the patient's face, the elder asked, "Should you now be healed, what will you do with your redeemed life?" Realizing the patient's situation made reflection and conversation unrealistic at the moment, the elder wisely squeezed the patient's hand lovingly and left. But the question certainly didn't leave the patient.

What about you? Every day is a gift. As a Christian, every day is redeemed by the grace of God. What will you do with the days you have left to show your thanksgiving to God for the time He has given you?

As for Christian healthcare, and being a practitioner of such, what about adopting a situation-appropriate variation of the question, "Should you be healed, what will you do with your life?" It is a question which will certainly open doors to real conversation and a better understanding of your patient.

Blessings to you and yours. Let's all make each day meaningful for ourselves and those around us. Most of all, let's make our days those of gratitude to God, expressed in service to Him through our Christian healthcare.

❧ A Reflection on Gratitude

My reflections this year have frequently taken me to the topic of gratitude. I've learned that I am not naturally a grateful person. I tend to expect things somehow are owed to me. Martin Luther was right when he observed all other sin sprung from the root of covetousness. When you think about it, that's the infantile attitude with which we are all born.

In Romans 1:18-21, the Apostle Paul warned that failure to look at creation with a sober, adult mind – a mind which has learned to be grateful to God, our creator – leaves us with a darkness in our hearts. Out of a dark heart flows a river of self-centered sin. So it behooves us to learn to see God at work in creation and our lives and to become grateful people.

Gratitude is a behavior learned over a lifetime. For me it has often been learned on the far side of surviving pain and struggle through the love and providence of God, family, and friends. Sometimes it is the stranger or the 'chance' encounter that prompts me to be grateful. Most often though, I learn the kind of gratefulness God desires me to have and express in the presence of God's grateful people. Paul the Apostle apparently felt the same way, for twice in the letter to the Colossians (2:6-7 and 3:16-17) he urged the church to teach one another to think about God and express gratitude.

> Gratitude is a learned behavior.

Express it in word, in deed, in psalm, in hymn and in spiritual songs.

In the name of Christ Jesus, our Messiah, be a grateful people.

Prayer

Cry out, articulate, or just groan;

you are asking God to change something.

May that change, first and foremost, be in you.

๛ Pray with Me

Jesus took Peter, James, and John to keep watch with and over Him during His anguished praying in the Garden of Gethsemane. They failed, falling asleep instead. So Jesus urged them to pray in order not to fall into temptation. They apparently failed at that twice. They neither kept watch with and over Jesus, or prayed with Him. They abandoned Him to His own horrible death, alone.

There are some pretty clear implications and applications for us as Christians in healthcare. May I point them out?

First, Jesus took the lead in praying. It was His severe situation. He expressed clearly to His companions how deeply troubled and distressed He was. If the disciples didn't reflexively begin praying with and for Him, at the very least, Jesus asked them to watch over Him as He prayed. If in the face of impending horror Jesus wanted to pray – needed to pray – we should see that prayer is vital at such times. Our patients, created in God's image and likeness, often want to pray too. Will you be there to help them? (See James 5:13-20)

Second, Jesus responded to the disciples falling asleep with an admonition to pray not to fall into temptation. Temptation to what? We can begin by seeing they were called to stand in a protective role for the Lord. Instead, however, sleep was their response, leaving Jesus unguarded. Jesus also knew they were weak in the flesh and would need spiritual bolstering at such a dire time.

Third, Jesus knew full well from prophesy that the sheep would be scattered and He would be abandoned ... something anyone in such desperate straits would fear. For as long as possible, He wanted to know they were with Him.

The Gethsemane account is written about Jesus and the three disciples, but it has been preserved to teach us what Jesus would want and do for someone else in such circumstances. When your patients face dire circumstances, will you stand with them and pray for them? Or will you fall asleep in the face of their anguish, effectively abandoning them?

❧ But What Should I Say?

Two of the most common questions I hear from Christians in healthcare when thinking about how to encourage their patients are: "What should I or can I pray with my Christian patient?" and "What if my patient isn't a Christian, but a Jew, Muslim, or of some other faith system?"

Let's consider the latter question first. All major monotheistic faith systems (Christian/Jewish/Muslim) accept the Old Testament as divinely inspired Scriptures. Most other faiths accept that scriptures exist and will listen to what yours say. So when in doubt, the best first place to go is the Old Testament. Given that, below is a suggestion for a passage to memorize or have handily marked for quick reference. It is one of those marked with the annotation, "Selah," which may loosely be understood as 'meditate on this thought.'

> *May the LORD be praised!*
> *Day after day He bears our burdens;*
> *God is our salvation.*   Selah
> *Our God is a God of salvation,*
> *And escape from death belongs to the*
> *LORD GOD.*
>
> Psalm 68:19-20

We can see why we should meditate on this passage. At first blush, it almost seems to open with a statement that will seem absurd to someone who is seriously ill. However, as we look at it, we praise God precisely because of the things the Lord does for us which are described in the text that follows: God bears our burdens daily (physical, in our soul, and spiritually), is willing and able to save us (sometimes temporally, always eternally), and, He is the overcomer and master of death.

112

Another meditative passage, which is a corollary to the idea of overcoming death, is Psalm 49:15: *But God will redeem my life from the power of Sheol* [the pit, the grave, death]*, for He will take me.*

As a Christian, you readily recognize that all of these promises found and continue to find their fulfillment in the Messiah, Jesus. If your patient asks, you can be quite explicit about that. But you don't have to start there. Begin by agreeing there is a God who is willing to walk all the way through your patient's care and illness with them. This brings hope and strength. The Holy Spirit will keep up the work you start.

To our initial question, how might you turn these passages into a prayer for or with your Christian patient? Ask God to be faithful to His promises. Here is a suggestion for how you might do that:

"God, thank you for promising to go with me through this illness. Thank you that I will be able to count on You to help me bear up every day. Thank you that You are able to bring complete healing, if that is Your will. Please guide my doctor towards that end. Thank you that as my God, no matter the final outcome of this illness, I know You desire to redeem me and take me to You forever. Amen."

ᔐ Confession & Healing Prayer

Please read James 5:13-20, a passage about anointing, prayer and healing. Let's look at the hub of these verses dealing with suffering, sickness, confession, remission of sins, and healing.

> *Therefore, confess your sins to one another and pray for one another, so that you may be healed. The urgent request of a righteous person is very powerful in its effect. Elijah was a man with a nature like ours; yet he prayed earnestly....*
>
> James 5:16-17a

Let's be very clear. Not all suffering or sickness is the result of sin or lostness. However, *sometimes* it is. The suffering or sickness may be in the body, in the soul (emotions, intellect, memories, and will), or both. *Sometimes* God will allow sickness as a tool for causing people with a still-gestational or infantile spirit to surrender their lives to Him and be born again spiritually or strengthen their spirit.

As a Christian providing healthcare, your following in Jesus' steps means you don't consider the body, soul, or spirit in isolation, but consider and care holistically for your patient's overall well-being. You may discover there are things in their lives which run counter to God's will and which should be confessed. If you ask the Holy Spirit for wisdom, He will show you how and when to have that conversation (James 1:5-8). Then you may want to pray to God for the healing of your patient. Here's where things get very personal to you.

James says the effectual prayers for healing come from the righteous; Elijah is given as an example. We might think Elijah, being a prophet, had a special holy hotline to God's ear.

114

But James says he was a man with *our same nature*. That means he, too, was a fallen sinner! So what was the key to Elijah's righteousness and, thus, the effectiveness of his prayers? Quite possibly the same key that God has given to every one of us as followers of Jesus: *If we confess our sins, He is faithful and righteous to forgive us our sins and to cleanse us from all unrighteousness* (1 John 1:8).

It comes down, at least in part, to the 'Speck and Log' parable (Matthew 7:3-5). It is good to take the speck out of someone's eye so they are healed and can see, but first make sure you have removed any logs in your own eye, so you can see with clarity to help them.

Before each shift where you will provide Christian care, pray and ask the Holy Spirit to identify any sin *you* need to confess. Genuinely confess it. Let God pluck the plank from your eye. Be declared righteous by Him. Then you may pray effective healing prayers for your patients.

ご Responding to Aggravation

Have you ever been made uncomfortable by a passage? I have. One that challenges me is this passage from Acts. I hope it challenges us all as Christians in healthcare.

> *Once, as we were on our way to prayer, a slave girl met us who had a spirit of prediction. She made a large profit for her owners by fortune-telling. As she followed Paul and us she cried out, "These men, who are proclaiming to you the way of salvation, are the slaves of the Most High God." And she did this for many days. But Paul was greatly aggravated and turning to the spirit, said, "I command you in the name of Jesus Christ to come out of her!" And it came out right away.*

Acts 16:16-18

Paul linked daily prayer with proclaiming the Good News that we can be saved from the penalty for our sins – freedom to the captives and a setting free of the oppressed (Luke 4:16-21). Do we daily link prayer with sharing the Good News? If not, do we think we can save people in our own strength and wisdom?

This pitiful girl was slave to men and demons. She was an example of the pitiful young people in our very midst who are being human-trafficked. Does it matter to us that this girl, or any one of our own patients, are trapped in bondage? Do we study enough clues that we might intervene as Jesus and Paul did to set them free?

Demons may be used by God to proclaim the truth about Jesus. If nobody will do it, even the rocks will cry out. Are we guilty of waiting for demons and rocks to do what we have been gifted, called, and placed to do? Why?

Paul was greatly aggravated. Was this because his prayer time was interrupted, his Gospel presentation derailed, or he just didn't like distractions? Maybe he was aggravated at the girl because she was yelling out that what Paul was proclaiming was true, but she wasn't following his advice. Maybe the girl had tried, but the demon was tenacious. (Jesus said that some will only come out after disciples get serious first about prayer and fasting for someone's deliverance). Have you ever encountered 'this girl' and instead of prayerfully asking the Holy Spirit to help you discern what is going on and how to set her free, you just got aggravated and left it at that?

Paul was ultimately shown to be aggravated at the demon, not the girl. He directed his healing strategy in the right direction, calling on Jesus Christ to deliver the girl from demonic control. Jesus set her free, but apparently He had been waiting for Paul to call on Him to do so. Has Jesus been waiting for you, too? Do you recognize that not every healthcare battle we fight involves flesh and blood? Some battles are certainly spiritual and call for you to offer a different level of care. Will you?

⁊ Preparing for Victory

In 1 Chronicles 14, the author recounts a story which first appeared in King David's biography recorded in 2 Samuel 5. The important points of the story are that while a situation may look familiar, and lull us into routine responses, David didn't do that. Instead David demonstrated his dependence on God for each new day or situation. He saw himself as God's agent. God got the credit for David's victories because David consulted with the Lord.

This year may *appear* as if it will be routine and mundane. However, just as the mercies of the Lord are new every morning, the Lord may very well have something new for you each day, regardless of the familiar package in which it comes. Are you looking for it, asking for discernment about it and thankful to receive it?

New Year's Day, birthdays, and anniversaries are wonderful opportunities for all of us in healthcare to reflect upon David's model for obtaining victory and gaining glory for God. Let's develop the life habit of asking God each day to open our eyes to what new opportunities are right in front of us. May we have the wisdom to ask God what *His* plans are for our day. May we charge when He says to;

> Be kind, for everyone you meet is fighting a hard battle.
>
> Ian MacLaren

wait patiently for the rustling of God's breath in the treetops when He says to wait; and, always be faithful to give Him the credit for the victories He uses us to obtain. May everyone with whom we come in contact share in the spoils that come to those who wait upon the Lord, even in the midst of the mundane or routine.

❧ Praying to Be an Agent of Grace

Thank you to Allan Samuelson, DDS and Clinical Associate Professor at UNC SOD, for reminding us what it is to be an agent of grace. He recommends this prayer by St. Francis for our consideration.

Lord, make me an instrument of Your peace;
Where there is hatred, let me sow love;
Where there is injury, pardon;
Where there is discord, harmony;
Where there is error, truth;
Where there is doubt, faith;
Where there is despair, hope;
Where there is darkness, light;
And where there is sadness, joy.

O Divine Master, grant that I may not so much seek
To be consoled as to console;
To be understood as to understand;
To be loved as to love.
For it is in giving that we receive;
It is in pardoning that we are pardoned;
And it is in dying that we are born to eternal life.

PERSEVERANCE

Then the Lord said to Paul in a night vision, "Don't be afraid, but keep on speaking and don't be silent. For I am with you, and no one will lay a hand on you to hurt you, because I have many people in this city."

Acts 18:9-10

The following night, the Lord stood by him and said, "Have courage! For as you have testified about Me in Jerusalem, so you must also testify in Rome."

Acts 23:11

❧ Lesson from a Sweaty Runner

The day before Dr. Al Weir, the CMDA President-Elect, spoke at the Triangle Christian Medical & Dental Association's spring retreat about how to make difficult decisions, he went for a late afternoon jog through the rural countryside. When he returned, sweat was pouring off him. He was seated on steps overlooking the lakefront, catching his breath, when I came upon him.

Looking up at me, he asked, "Do you run?"

Thinking from a purely physical perspective, I replied, "Not if I can help it. I've never seen a runner smiling while they run. Only when they're done."

Grinning a bit, Dr. Weir responded, "Yeah, about two hours later, when the endorphins kick in, then it is worth it."

It occurred to me that Dr. Weir must run everywhere he goes, at least one of his motivations being that after the hard part, later, comes the pleasure and reward. He comes from the 'old school' that delayed gratification is gratification that has so much value it gives us the motivation to persevere through hardship.

Dr. Weir's physical model has much to say to us spiritually – it is much like the physical and spiritual lessons of the Apostle Paul, 2,000 years ago. Like Dr. Weir, Paul's spiritual running had many venues. Paul's rewards came after a year and a half of ministry in Corinth. Later Paul spent three years in Ephesus, three months in the synagogue followed by a year and a half in the lecture hall. He talked among the Jews and Gentiles alike.

Sometimes the lay of the land was fairly easy downhill, but it had lots of steep climbing against fierce resistance too. Paul also wore diverse running shoes at different times. He taught as a tentmaker, returned for follow up visits, sent emissaries to give and get updates, and he wrote lofty letters of encouragement and admonition. No matter what the terrain or trial, Paul kept running his spiritual race to teach and proclaim the goodness of Jesus Christ to anyone who would listen.

If you are a Christian in healthcare, either practicing or studying to practice, the questions you have to answer are, "Will I start (or keep) running? If I run the race to which God has called me – to be His ambassador of reconciliation – will I endure over the hard trails and through frequent trials? Will I fit my shoes to the situation so I stand the best chance of successfully finishing the race? Will I learn to appreciate the valuable rewards of oft-delayed gratification?"

Dr. Weir came with two hours' worth of wisdom and visuals to teach us an orderly method for making godly decisions in healthcare and life. Little did he know his runner's sweat spoke volumes long before he began his lecture. I've decided to keep on running the race, despite the pain, in order to receive the God-promised heavenly gain. Will you?

ல் Joe & Nic

Healthcare education, research, and practice have become a huge community, employing thousands of people. While everyone involved has a role to play, clearly there is a subset within the community that leans academically in penchant and focus. There is nothing wrong whatsoever with that. The form and future of medicine is often seen and shaped years in advance by women and men of such nature.

If you happen to be such a person and a Christian as well – for the two are not mutually exclusive, despite the protestations of some – you face challenges which may make you feel like an unwelcome minority. In fact, you might actually be so. Therefore, in a research environment that is highly competitive, and that demands grant funding, cooperation from administrations, and publication for promotion, you might be tempted to suppress signs of your carefully considered faith in Jesus. It is easier – for a while, anyhow – to travel a path of reduced resistance, questions, and conflict.

However, as an adopted child of God, you aren't called to a path of ease. Jesus told us that in this world, because of His Name and our association with Him, we would have tribulation and trouble. Life as a follower of Christ would be attended by trials. It was in just such trials that all four Gospels introduce us to two fellow academics: Joseph of Arimathea and Nicodemus (Nic-at-night). The latter Jesus called a 'teacher of Israel,' (likely a scribe). The former was a member of the Sanhedrin. Their stories in the Gospels are worth reviewing.

Jesus' teaching and actions were highly disruptive and disturbing to the order the chief priests, elders, scribes and Sanhedrin had established and maintained. Mark's Gospel records at least three times that the establishment looked for a way to seize and kill Jesus. John 7:45-52 and John 19:38 make plain that in those days to be an academic and a disciple of Jesus was politically and personally risky too. In a sense Joe and Nic are the Christian academic's archetypes.

There are several lessons and encouragements Christian academics can derive from the stories of Joe and Nic.

- First, there is nothing wrong or sinful about being gifted by God to be thinkers and leaders. Every culture and community needs such people.

- Second, Joe and Nic didn't take Jesus at face value. They observed, listened, and asked questions. As a result of studying their subject – Jesus and His claims – they found Him to be the Way to the Kingdom of God they had been seeking. It is okay for you to critically consider your faith, as well.

- Third, because of their considered convictions, at the critical moment of the crucifixion, they stepped forward to serve God by caring for Jesus' body. Out of the night, into the light.

Their legacy is yours to carry on. Will you?

↪ Standing on Great Shoulders

Have you ever been in a situation where someone who doesn't know any better belittles your faith in God by claiming that the Bible was written by ignorant or superstitious, myth-telling people? Who would foolishly believe and put their trust in such writings? Here is a quick thought you might want to share with them.

Moses, the author of the Pentateuch, *was educated in all the wisdom of the Egyptians and was powerful in his speech and actions* (Acts 7:22). That would make him an engineer, architect, or astronomer, and someone able to read and write.

Of King Solomon it is said,

> God gave Solomon wisdom, very great insight, and understanding as vast as the sand on the seashore. Solomon's wisdom was greater than the wisdom of all the people of the East, greater than all the wisdom of Egypt. ...People came from everywhere, sent by every king on earth who had heard of his wisdom, to listen to Solomon's wisdom.
>
> 1 Kings 4:29-34

Daniel, arguably the most politically influential Jew in ancient history, as well as a comprehensively accurate prophet, was a

> young [man] without any physical defect, good-looking, suitable for instruction in all wisdom, knowledgeable, perceptive and capable of serving in the king's palace – and [able to learn] the Chaldean language and literature. ... Daniel also understood visions and dreams of every kind. ... In

126

*every matter of wisdom and understanding that
the king consulted [Daniel] about, he found [Dan-
iel] 10 times better than all the diviner-priests and
mediums in his entire kingdom.*

Daniel 1:4, 17a, 20

And who can argue with the intellect and rhetorical skills of
the Apostle Paul? The Apostle Peter said of Paul's writings,

*Also, regard the patience of our Lord as an oppor-
tunity for salvation, just as our dear brother Paul
has written to you according to the wisdom given
to him. He speaks about these things in all his letters in which there are some matters that are hard
to understand. The untaught and unstable twist
them to their own destruction, as they also do with
the rest of Scriptures.*

2 Peter 3:15-16

When your faith is challenged as unreasonable and standing on shaky intellectual ground, stand your ground confidently. In the power of the Holy Spirit, great minds
recorded and exposed the Law, natural law, political law,
and Jesus' life – the grace-based point of all laws – to reveal
God. Your faith stands on the shoulders of some of history's
greatest minds, inspired by God Himself.

‿ Right of Conscience Decades Later

I attended the Voice of Christian Doctors Media Workshop at CMDA headquarters. The leadership team trained us to educate the public effectively on important medical issues through print, radio, and TV. We are all called to be salt and light. Christians in healthcare have an abundance of both to dispense, if we will speak out through media in a way the public can taste and see.

The subject of the right of conscience for healthcare workers came up as one topic needing salt and light. We were made aware of an article published in 1949 on conscience and healthcare. If you've not read the chilling article by Leo Alexander, MD, "Medical Science Under Dictatorship," do so. The article sounds an alarm that those in healthcare with a conscience may be the final line of patient defense against state-mandated or corporate-sponsored killing.

> Those in healthcare with a conscience may be the final line of patient defense against state-mandated or corporate-sponsored killing.

Alexander's observations about differing cultures and physician communities cast the Dutch and American medical communities in pretty good light – rooted in moral and ethical soil. This was in contrast to a medical community that had surrendered conscience to take up a politico-philosophical worldview that "what is useful is right." Who determined what was useful and, therefore, right? No longer God, but government. Physicians with this new worldview became prime instructors and instruments for making things 'right' (economically, politically, and socially), resulting in human horrors on a previously unimaginable scale.

Now the Dutch medical community leads the world in promoting physician-assisted death and physician-inflicted killing. In the United States, federal takeover of healthcare for social and economic reasons is bureaucratically crushing healthcare-related conscience protesters. Individual states like Oregon have traded paying to alleviate suffering through good medical care with paying physicians to kill those who suffer. It is more 'cost effective' and 'compassionate.'

Alexander noted that utilitarian philosophies regarding healthcare as a tool rather than a treatment took root as soon as enough people in medicine started believing they were able to judge which lives were not worth living, as opposed to holding a conviction that all life is equally valuable. It soon became 'normal' to let practitioners, not God, dictate who lived and died when external powers (such as government, societies, practice boards, employers, and colleagues) used fear of fines, ostracism, and unemployment to coerce conformity to the new paradigm.

For patients to maintain trust in their practitioner, they must be sure she or he has only their best interest at heart, including healing of their body, soul, and spirit. To keep that trust, it is incumbent upon practitioners to vigorously and loudly fight to practice with their God-given conscience at their core. **Surrendering the right of conscience is surrendering being trustworthy to our patients and puts everyone in grave danger.**

ও Guard Your God-Given Rights

With the signing of the Declaration of Independence, our Founding Fathers made clear that all people should be free to exercise their God-given rights to life, liberty, and the pursuit of happiness. The first right in our Bill of Rights made explicit that government may not infringe upon life, liberty, and the pursuit of happiness by interfering with our personal practice of religion, whether in speech or deed.

As Christian healthcare practitioners who live in the United States of America, we should be thanking God often that we live in a land where, in principle at least, we not only have these rights, but in our calling we can daily strive – in speech and deed – to enable all people we serve to also enjoy their God-given rights. What an amazing privilege!

Why say, "in principle at least?" Well, as privileged scientists who thrive on evidence, let's recall the important and very practical lesson of the Second Law of Thermodynamics, paraphrased as, "any system which does not have energy applied to it, will devolve into chaos and coldness." Our rights are spelled out as part of a system, which involves not only the written principles, but also the people as the guardians and the government as defender of those principles. Since the rules can't rewrite themselves, and if the rule-defenders choose to ignore rather than defend them, then the only energy left to keep the system

> May we think of freedom, not as the right to do as we please, but as the opportunity to do what is right.
>
> Peter Marshall

working must come from the guardian-people to whom the rules apply. That is us.

So let's thank God that our nation was built upon a foundation of recognizing and protecting our God-given rights. Let's also, however, thank Him by applying our energy to guard those rights. In so doing, we not only demonstrate we are citizens of America *and* of God's kingdom, but we protect our ability to serve through healing our fellow human beings in all stages of their life, so they too may pursue liberty and happiness.

ENDURANCE

You have demonstrated you have the capacity to endure.

Nobody gets to practice healthcare without first proving that.

But will you choose to run the race

God has marked out for you?

Will you continue to run that race so as to win?

ও Meeting Together

... and let us consider [thoughtfully] how we may
encourage one another to love and to do good
deeds, not forsaking our meeting together [as be-
lievers for worship and instruction], as is the habit
of some, but encouraging one another; and all the
more [faithfully] as you see the day [of Christ's re-
turn] approaching.

Hebrews 10:24-25, AMP

According to Dr. Richard Swenson, of some 800,000 physicians in the US, approximately 300,000 are burned out. That doesn't include residents, who at one medical training center, for example, reported burnout rates of 44%-77%! Many doctors have lost enthusiasm for what they do, are at least inwardly dismissive of patients, and wish they could retire or find another line of work. They don't see what they do as making a real difference anymore and wonder why they keep doing it. Burnout also infects allied health-care team members, multiplying its negative influence.

Almost any one of us can find reasons and excuses for our frustration with what medicine has become and how far it has been jolted off the cornerstone ideals of service, caring, and, hopefully, healing. Yet, as Christians in healthcare, we have the ability to build and maintain our practice on a solid, unshakable Rock – the Chief Cornerstone – who is Christ Jesus. Yes, medicine now seems to be tottering on shifting sand. However, if we adopt the eternal perspective of God, we see our vocation as medical ambassadors of reconciliation cannot be shaken or moved. It is enduringly meaningful.

When we join together to pray for, encourage, instruct, admonish, and bless one another, we renew and increase our ability to endure through the hard times and difficult changes. We are reminded not to look around at our situation but upwards to our Savior and inwards to our source of strength, the Holy Spirit. Together we remind one another of our eternal purpose for being Christians in healthcare. Whether teaching each other how to bring hope to the hopeless, or standing side-by-side, statewide, against Death on Demand thinking, let's be faithful to gather together.

> *Therefore, since we also have such a large cloud of witnesses surrounding us, let us lay aside every weight and the sin that so easily ensnares us. Let us run with endurance the race that lies before us, keeping our eyes on Jesus, the source and perfecter of our faith, who for the joy that lay before Him endured a cross and despised the shame and has sat down at the right hand of God's throne. ...consider Him who endured such hostility from sinners against Himself, so that you won't grow weary and lose heart. ...Therefore, since we are receiving a kingdom that cannot be shaken, let us hold on to grace. By it, we may serve God acceptably, with reverence and awe, for our God is a consuming fire.*
>
> Hebrews 12:1-3, 28-29

෨ Walking Together

A trip with my family gave me the opportunity to escape from my work cocoon, spread my wings, and freshly experience life on the streets. I was struck by an observation. Many groups of two to four people walking the boulevards, riding trains, or sitting side by side in airports were apparently affiliated with one another yet seemed disassociated. These folks, free to engage with one another as they journeyed, were in their own cocoons, formed by pocket-sized colored boxes in their hands and white wires hanging out of their ears.

Such sights, over and over, reminded me of how our culture is changing so rapidly. On so many fronts, the truth proclaimed by the prophet Amos is being sorely tested. *Can two walk together without agreeing to meet?* (Amos 3:3) In my meditation on what I was seeing, I realized that even in our own community of Christians in healthcare, we are testing Amos' message from God. Can that be a good thing? *Selah.*

> We must agree to meet and walk together, mutually supporting one another. That remains God's truth.

Relax. This isn't a screed against technology, podcasts, etc. These things are, in many ways, capacity multipliers helping us extend our reach and resources to do good. Instead, this is a call to each of us to beware of isolation, including the isolation that takes place in a busy practice or classroom, surrounded by people all day long. We risk becoming just so many Christian healthcare cocoons.

Amos wasn't the only one warning of the dangers of isolation. Solomon also addressed this.

> *Iron sharpens iron, and one man sharpens another.*
>
> Proverbs 27:17

> *Two are better than one because they have a good reward for their efforts. For if either falls, his companion can lift him up; but pity the one who falls without another to lift him up. Also, if two lie down together, they can keep warm; but how can one person alone keep warm? And if someone overpowers one person, two can resist him. A cord of three strands is not easily broken.*
>
> Ecclesiastes 4:9-12

As Christians in healthcare, we are not only adopted children in God's family, we are part of a profoundly privileged tribe within this family. We are the ambassadors for Christ with the unique ability to follow in Jesus' footsteps by simultaneously healing bodies, teaching souls, and speaking to spirits. Our tribe has a high calling and huge responsibility.

In our increasingly secularized, utilitarian, pluralistic, and complex culture, remaining faithful and true to our highest calling – using healthcare as a vehicle for ministry in Christ's name – is getting harder and harder. In order to fulfill our mission to minister to our peers, colleagues, and patients, we need each other as mutual instruments of edification and encouragement.

Ideally, we find ways to agree to meet in person. Alternatively, when schedules preclude face-to-face, we leverage technology to meet. Somehow though, we must agree to meet and walk together, mutually supporting one another. That remains God's truth.

❧ Professional Salvation

Cardiologist Sandeep Jauhar titled his essay in the *Wall Street Journal* on 29 August, 2014, "Why Doctors Are Sick of Their Profession." He catalogues a long list of complaints about circumstances and factors that have robbed many in healthcare of joy and motivation. As he describes it, practitioners are in a state of "malaise." Dr. Jauhar cries the lament of a battle-weary soldier being pursued by multiple enemies of ideals, fulfillment, and hope.

Just when the reader is about to abandon all hope, Dr. Jauhar makes an attempt to redeem the healthcare profession from its enemies. He is worth quoting here, not because what he says is correct, but because as Christians in healthcare we can empathize with what he seeks but fails to find.

> "In the end, the problem is one of resilience. American doctors need an internal compass to navigate the changing landscape of our profession. For most doctors, this compass begins and ends with their patients. In surveys, most physicians – even the dissatisfied ones – say the best part of their jobs is taking care of people. I believe this is the key to coping with the stresses of contemporary medicine: identifying what is important to you, what you believe in, and what you will fight for.

> "What's most important to me as a doctor, I've learned, are the human moments. Medicine is about taking care of people in their most vulnerable states and making yourself

somewhat vulnerable in the process. …Ultimately, this is the best hope for our professional salvation."

Dr. Jauhar may have struck truth when he connected coping with believing something is important enough to fight for. But he'll never slay the enemies of his professional satisfaction doing it the way he describes. First, notice his compass is internal. It will always, therefore, be subject to emotions, fatigue, whim, and opinion. His needle sits on a bent spindle. Second, his loadstone is the ever-moving target of other people. Elsewhere Jauhar complains people don't give doctors enough respect. Dr. Jauhar's prescription won't lead to "professional salvation" (a curious choice of words).

David, a man also very skilled and called to a lofty profession as King of Israel, offers the way to find professional salvation. At times it seemed heaven and earth conspired to destroy David. He, too, could be downcast. Yet his famous words (Psalm 23) begin and end by describing the essentials that allowed him to continue steadfast in his vocation.

First, David didn't look to himself or other people to find what he needed. *The LORD is my shepherd; there is nothing I lack* (Psalm 23:1).

Second, David recognized enemies and trials will come and go, but *Only goodness and faithful love will pursue me all the days of my life, and I will dwell in the house of the LORD as long as I live* (Psalm 23:6; see also Psalm 27:4-6 – the victory found dwelling in God's presence).

Circumstances and the enemy of our soul may conspire to kill, steal, or destroy our happiness. The solution isn't found in the inconstancy and fallibility of humanity. It is in knowing and abiding in the Good Shepherd, Jesus, who meets our every need for personal and professional salvation.

ᖇ A Thought about Independence

Have you observed that in declaring our independence from Great Britain, we *did not* declare our independence from God and each other? In the season of our founding, we recognized God in His loving wisdom providentially involves Himself in the affairs of humanity, including founding a great nation like ours. And we recognized that a nation is made up of "we the people."

So in this contemporary age when 'personal autonomy' is a dominant buzzword over healthcare practice, leading as it inevitably has to state-endorsed and doctor-enforced death, maybe this is the right time to remind ourselves of the biblical concept of independence.

Please indulge me as I borrow from *Matters of Life and Death* (InterVarsity Press, Nottingham, 2009) by our esteemed colleague Dr. John Wyatt. His words are wise.

> "Human beings are not self-explanatory. We derive our meaning from outside ourselves, from God, in whose image we are made. We are not autonomous individuals, constantly creating ourselves by the decisions and choices we make.
>
> "For a society penetrated by liberal individualism as ours is, this concept is peculiar, nonsensical, even outrageous. Yet the biblical revelation stresses our creaturely dependence [See Job 10:8-12, 34:14-15 and Jeremiah 10:23].
>
> "God has not made us as independent individuals sprouting up like mushrooms in a

field. He has put us in families, locked together in mutual dependence. Not only are we designed to depend on God; we are also designed to depend on one another. We come into the world as helpless infants, totally dependent on another's love and care. ...Then we go through a phase of our lives when other people depend on us. ...And then most of us will end our physical lives totally dependent on the love and care of others. We will need other people to feed us, protect us, and wipe our bottoms. And this is not a terrible, degrading inhuman reality. It's part of the design. It is an integral part of the narrative of a person's life."

Of course nobody would advocate the degrading of any person. Every individual is uniquely and specially created in God's image and likeness, and is, therefore, supremely valuable. As part of God's image, people also have the capacity for making choices. Therefore, we have a responsibility to bring salt and light to our patient's souls. That may well include teaching them that 'personal autonomy' is not a historically understood concept, and leads to choices which are potentially harmful to the patient and counter to your deeply held beliefs about what is in the patient's best interest.

Let's carefully consider the difference between independence from tyranny and independence from God and one another. We should encourage the former. We should discourage the latter.

❧ Building the Kingdom Together

I want to encourage us with points related to our role and location as Christian health care practitioners and students. These truths come from Nehemiah's description of rebuilding the walls of Jerusalem, recorded in Nehemiah 3 and 4. Please read them before this note of encouragement.

First, every gate had a name and that name can be related to some key point of the Gospel. All of life, whatever we are doing, ought to be lived as a testimony to the one and only Gospel which saves. That includes our studies and practices of medicine.

Second, there was plenty of wall for everyone to build. We don't need to envy or worry about someone else's place or role in healthcare. God has a role and a place for *us*. We are in it now. Let's appreciate that.

Third, God knew the names of every family who was at their place, doing their task. He also knew and called out those who *weren't*. Are you serving the Lord in your place? Even if it is not glamorous, God sees, knows, and is recording these things in preparation for rewarding you. He also knows those who aren't about the Master's business, but only about their own (1 Corinthians 3:5-15).

Fourth, everyone was expected to participate as part of God's people: priests, administrators, goldsmiths, apothecaries (hey, you pharmacists), retailers, women, and men. Everyone was eligible to serve God, regardless of their vocation or gender. The same goes for Christians in healthcare.

Fifth, everyone managed to carry both a trowel and a sword. It might have been easier to hold one or the other, but we are not called to easy. We are in a spiritual battle every bit as much as we are in a physical battle against pain, suffering, disease and decay. We can and must wield the trowel of our practice with skill *and* wield the sword of the Spirit, which is the Word of God.

May God give you a vision of yourself as one who is serving Him and building alongside others in your place of study or practice. May you recognize you are valuable to Him. He knows what you are doing even in the hard times, and is laying up eternal rewards for your faithfulness to the task of rebuilding that which is broken before you every day.

ぞ The Principle of Two-by-Two

- It was not good to be alone, so the role of helpmates appeared in Genesis 2.

- Every soulish creation that entered Noah's ark to survive the global flood of judgment entered the ark as part of a pair at the minimum ...no solo actors in Genesis 7.

- Solomon – the wisest man ever until Jesus – expounded on the advantages of small groups of two or three in Ecclesiastes 4:9-12.

- On very rare occasions, God sent out prophets alone. How many people can you think of who went astray or despaired or became depressed – even in God's service – in part because of their sense of aloneness or having nobody to listen to them?

- Poor Job. In his time of troubles, where was anyone to help him stand, keep him warm, hear his heart, or fend off Satan's attacks?

- By the time of the New Testament, we see that Jesus virtually never sent any of His disciples out alone (Ananias in Damascus or Philip on the desert road being exceptions to the rule). Even for an intellectual giant like Paul, God 'thorned' his prowess so that he would have to travel everywhere with a supportive partner.

Those of us in healthcare tend to be self-starters, intellectually astute, and hard workers. We have many people counting on us in life-changing ways. We are generally well compensated financially or through praise and approbation for the work we do. To outsiders, sometimes including our pastors, we appear to have it made. People think we don't face trials like 'mere mortals' do.

Now, don't get me wrong. As Christians who have a good grasp of Scripture, we don't think more highly of ourselves then we ought, we know our brokenness and repent of our sins, and, we walk before our Savior and Lord with humility and reverence. But many of us also recognize that people often look upon us with a certain sense of awe, respect, and belief we have it all together. Therein lies a seed of isolation leading to frustration, despair, and burnout. Does anyone really understand our struggles and our humanity? Who can stand alongside us?

> People think we don't face trials like 'mere mortals' do.

The clue to answering that question lies in Jesus' way with His disciples. Jesus paired or tripled up people who not only had a calling to serve God, but also a gender, community and/or trade affinity. Binding together these kinds of small groups He sent out wonder-working teachers, preachers, and healers. *Together* they rose above trials (see Matthew 4, 9-10; Mark 6; Luke 10; and Acts 4).

Based on the biblical examples, we ought to prayerfully and practically bear one another's burdens as nobody else can. We must mutually counter isolation and create mechanisms whereby we may stand with one another.

May you see the value of building these relationships. May the Holy Spirit give you the vision and inspiration to stand beside brothers and sisters as we share the privileged position of healthcare ministers.

∂ Will You Let Jesus Teach You Rest?

Healthcare ministers are in a privileged position to walk in the footsteps of Jesus, but they are not immune to growing weary, burdened, and feeling heavy laden. Getting to know and pray with so many of you, I can testify that there are some common challenges we face, even if our settings and specifics vary.

First, we sign up for more than we can actually do *well*. So we build up an internal pressure from being self-driven and then find ourselves ricocheting from one task to another.

Second, our situations and circumstances – family, finances, practices, and even our own health – are in flux. In response, we may fear, resist, or resent changes imposed on us.

Third, many of us enjoy being part of a good church, a loving small group, and/or having a ministry outside work. That's not the same, however, as having a comforting and encouraging relationship with other Christians in healthcare who best understand our struggles. Even more important, nothing substitutes for daily time with Christ, who gave us this healthcare calling (1 Corinthians 4:7).

In Matthew 11:20-30, Jesus offers a real solution for those who are burdened, heavy laden, and weary. He calls us to come receive rest *His* way, through a tripartite plan.

Use your spiritual eyes.

God is with you. He is with your every circumstance. He is still in the miracle-working business as a sign of His ever present concern for you. Don't rely upon fleshly eyes, which only see situations in dark grays of habit or past experiences. This is worse than dead-end thinking. Instead, envision the bright hues of new possibilities with God.

Don't be enamored by your own wisdom or authority, thinking you are God.

You were adopted by God to become His child, through a childlike faith He gave you. Trust that God, your *Abba* Father, has the real power and authority over all things – even the frustrating externals imposed upon you. Nothing can happen to you that God can't remake for something good or useful. (Think of Jonah or Job as examples.) Humble yourself and, if necessary, abdicate. In faith let God the King sit on the throne of your life.

Jesus is calling, but are we listening to what He is saying?

Elsewhere God calls the weary to walk beside still waters, to lie down in green pastures and to dine with Him. In this passage though, Jesus' promise isn't to give us physical rest. Neither is it to salvation and spiritual highs. It is to hear Him teach our souls (emotions, intellect, memories, and will) to think like Him so that we can live in a state of rest. His offer to us is a renewed mind which doesn't inflict us with stress. We are not worn down by the externals. We can live an abundant life out from under the thinking which robs us of the joy of our salvation and service.

Give yourself to Christ's call to be delivered from your burden(s). One could say He gave us one day in seven to rest our bodies and reflect in community on spiritual blessings. The other six days at least, He offers to teach us His way to have a rested mind. Also, please make a point of praying for and coming alongside your fellow Christians in healthcare who are burdened. God wants to help them, too. Won't you go with them to hear Jesus?

ಿ Do Not Lose Sight of the Obvious

Have you ever wondered where your glasses were? Your car keys? You start searching, keep searching, and finally ask someone. They smile that knowing smile and tell you, "They're on your head" or "In your hand." Sometimes things are so obvious that we somehow fail to recognize them. If that can happen to us in the physical realm, I suspect it can happen spiritually too.

In 2 Timothy, the Apostle Paul spent a great deal of time speaking about the spiritually obvious to a person who was losing sight of it. Paul was warning Timothy that he was in grave danger of neglecting God's call on his life, if not even quitting on it all together. The pressures and distractions of the past and present were blinding Timothy to the real and enduring future for himself and humanity. Chapter 3 of this epistle states this most starkly in a contrast of two thoughts.

> Sometimes things are so obvious that we somehow fail to recognize them.

The first thought is that the way of the earthly, temporary, human-wisdom controlled world is towards entropy – increasing coldness, chaos, and ultimately, dissolution. Things increasingly will seem to be coming apart.

The second, contrasting, thought is that the eternal, enduring, orderly path to a future of light, hope, and power is found in believing and obeying God's Word, which points to every person's need for the salvation and lordship of Jesus Christ. Paul was writing to Timothy, a beloved spiritual son, to stabilize him in his wavering or, possibly, to snatch him from an impending fall (see Jude 20-23).

148

Many of us may, like Timothy, be losing sight of the lost and dying people in our sphere of influence and we may be wavering in our assurance that we have been called as agents of grace to share the love and truth of the Gospel with them. The 'wisdom' of this world, the pressures of our studies, and the distractions of our professional and home lives are just as capable of causing us to buckle in our stand on God's Word and thus weaken in our commitment to God's call.

2 Timothy 3 shows us that the dividing line between entropy and enduring is whether we really trust God's Word as wholly reliable, inerrant, and infallible – everything we need to lead a godly life. He makes clear that the 'spectacles' we need to restore and maintain our vision of the obvious is ongoing trust in God's Word, pointing to Jesus. If we are not confident that God's Word is fully adequate to stand up to and overcome the wisdom of this world, we'll not be confident to share it with others who need to hear it in order to come to faith in Jesus Christ as their own Savior and Lord.

We ought to praise God He loves us enough to send people to us who can point out to us when we are losing sight of the obvious value and importance of trusting God's Word and the faith it births. Having such people speak encouragement and truth to us is part of our being discipled. We do well to listen, take heed, and act when God sends someone to us to build up our confidence in God's Word as the fountainhead of the faith leading to eternal life and a godly walk. We make serious errors neglecting such gifts of counsel for optional seasons of worldly pleasures or bowls of red lentils (see Hebrews 11:24-27; Genesis 25:29-34).

❧ Discernment

I had the privilege of fellowship with two Christian health-care practitioners. They were ministers doing very different things in very different settings. They clearly had the joy of the Lord in their lives. Yet they both spoke along a common theme: they needed discernment regarding their circumstances. One was happy where he practiced but now had a hint God might be moving him to a new situation. The other was in a setting where there was little happiness and was considering moving to another setting – only to have a sense he was being called to stay put. So what was God doing, where was He leading, and how should they follow Him? These were their questions.

Notice they were doing the right thing in the way they were asking those questions. God was at the heart of each question, not the happiness of the person asking. They demonstrated a right attitude with their questions, and their challenge then became how to discern the answers.

First, wisdom and victory can come from seeking the counsel of advisers (e.g., Proverbs 15:22). *Who should be our counselors and advisers?* If we take God's Word seriously, then we recognize that regardless of our specific vocation, we all share certain common and eternal things: we are of one body and share the same Holy Spirit, are called to the same hope, have the same faith in and are likewise baptized into the same Lord Jesus Christ, belong to the same God and Father; and, we share the mind of Christ (Ephesians 4:4-5; 1 Corinthians 2:16b). Who better to seek advice from about discerning God's leading than from those who already share so much with us in God *and* who also have an affinity with us through our similar vocations?

Second, it is important to be building relationships with such people on an ongoing basis, for we don't know when we may need their help or one of them might need our counsel. That's one major reason we so strongly encourage participation in Christian healthcare organizations. Here are people not only willing to come alongside you in counsel, but to go with you in prayer to God's throne, seeking discernment for you in your situation.

Third, will your decisions contribute to building on the foundation of proclaiming Christ crucified (silver, gold, and precious stones) or building on the shifting sands of happiness (wood, hay, and straw)? Paul and Peter encourage us to focus on building what will last, not on things which will one day burn up (1 Corinthians 3:10-15; 1 Peter 3:7-10).

May God show us that we as Christian healthcare ministers need one another, both in a horizontal peer-to-peer manner and a vertical mentoring relationship. As the pace of change and consequence in healthcare accelerates, so too does our need to share godly counsel and encouragement with one another. May the Lord aid each of us in building relationships which will help us discern His leading for our lives and the lives of those we counsel.

Discernment is not

knowing the difference

between right and wrong.

It is knowing the difference between

right and almost right.

Charles H. Spurgeon

✑ Three Keys for Enduring to Victory

> *For whatever was written in the past was written for our instruction, so that we may have hope through endurance and through the encouragement from the Scriptures. Now may the God who gives endurance and encouragement allow you to live in harmony with one another, according to the command of Christ Jesus, so that you may glorify the God and Father of our Lord Jesus Christ with a united mind and voice.*
>
> Romans 15:4-6

The Apostle Paul was fixated on enduring to the end. Maybe it came from his love of sports, from which he often drew metaphors about the spiritual 'race' we are running. Even in this passage, we can see Paul alluding to three keys to enduring to the end and being victorious: have a playbook, be part of a cohesive team, and listen to the coach in order to please him.

Have a Playbook

The Holy Spirit and the authors were writing Scripture for us. They had a very specific purpose: to encourage us to endure all the way to the end of the race. Sometimes the encouragement comes from observing what saints of the past did well, or shouldn't have done. Other times we are encouraged to avoid Satan's schemes and traps. Occasionally we are commanded. The playbook comes in many forms. I happen to use book, audio, smartphone, and the five-year Bible study of the Thru-the-Bible app (http://ttb.org/programs/broadcasts-podcasts), as my schedule requires. The key is to study the Word of God. It is our playbook.

Be a Team Player

Healthcare is a team sport. So is the Christian faith, as demonstrated by Jesus dying to birth the church, which He now coaches. If we are going to effectively minister through Christian healthcare, we need to be part of a team of Christians ministering through medicine. We need each other to help us finish strong.

Listen to and Please the Coach

In a very real sense, what God wants to do is communicated to us through the principles and many of the practices recorded in Scripture. Doing as a team what we are coached to do brings God glory.

Being a Christian in healthcare is not easy. We need to access and apply the tools God has given us to endure to the end of the race. Are you using the keys to run the distance and finish strong?

౨ Out of the Mouths of Geniuses

While we were in Germany, my beloved and I had the privilege of sharing an intimate dinner with a gentleman who earned a PhD in pharmaceutical chemistry and is now the head of product development for a major global concern. If I was focused on our relative intellects, I would have been ashamed to open my mouth in his presence. But I knew I was on a divine appointment to expose him and his wife to the love of Jesus. The spirit of fear was replaced with one of boldness and love.

When He asked what I did for a living, I had the chance to tell him how very blessed by God I was to be a follower of Jesus and minister in a variety of ways to women and men in healthcare. I teach them about sharing the love of Jesus, fellowship with them, give them a safe place to speak of their concerns and pains, and pray for them.

I wish each of you could have seen his response, for words fail me in describing it. He was moved. To paraphrase him, 'People have priests, patients have chaplains, but doctors? We don't have such a thing as this in Germany. I think we need it, too.'

We are part of a special situation in which we have encouraging fellowship with one another through CMDA nationally and in our local campus chapters and ministry groups here in North Carolina. Let's recognize that, as this gentleman did, and eagerly participate in it.

Overcoming

Your mission to provide Christian healthcare

may not always go the way you planned.

"Houston, we have a problem."

But there's a whole team of people

standing with and pulling for you.

"Failure is not an option."

ᔚ Overcoming "Yeah, but ..."

Please forgive me if I have somehow led any of you to believe that by virtue of the fact I bear the title "Pastor" I have had an airy-fairy, pristine, and trouble free life. Thus, I cannot possibly understand your challenges and fears as Christians in healthcare. Allow me to correct the record.

My childhood was not joyful abandon and fun. I was bent hard toward 'life is about duty.' I operated for decades trying to be responsible, in control, and a perfectionist. I lived in the fear of failure and disappointing others. On the Bust the Commandments exam, I have scored a solid 90%. In a couple youthful fits of rage, I came close to making that 100%. I know how to sin openly and secretly as well as the next guy.

Having become a follower of Jesus at almost the same time as entering the vocation of emergency medical services, I felt like Mercury's winged staff squeezed in coils between two dueling serpents – picture a caduceus. On one side of the helix, 'duty' demanded I evangelize the whole world. On the other side of the helix were the smothering coils under which I worked: society's devolving political correctness; federal, state and accreditation regulations; employer policies; and fear of offending peers or patients. All of these threatened to choke out my light. So I lived for years with a crushing sense of conflict, guilt, and even fear for my job – my livelihood.

So when I share with other Christians in healthcare about how privileged they are to walk in the footsteps of our Savior and Lord Jesus in our vocations, and the responses come back, "Yeah, but..." I empathize with you. I was there, too. I really do get it.

But God

Jesus never meant for us to live life under the whip. Jesus came to set us free, not flog us! If we do not experience the joy of our salvation, but instead feel stressed about living our lives as new creations in Christ before all people, it may be because we do not recognize the devilish schemes being perpetrated on us.

How many of us have hidden the following caricature of the Great Commission in our hearts? "As you go, get in their face, stuff a Four Spiritual Laws tract in their hand, and drag them down the Roman Road." Even if we have not, the question this commandment raises but does not answer is, "How do I do that, Lord? Making disciples, baptizing and teaching is a long-term process and I have so little time with my peers or patients." Without an answer to that question, we sit in painful paralysis, afraid of making a big mistake with the very first step. The answer to the question is found in three other passages.

Acts 2:46-47 – Solomon's Colonnade *and* House to House

It is vital we recognize that we live life in public spaces and small, more private and intimate communities. Public spaces are where we make proclamations. Dialogue and discipleship lend themselves much more to small groups. Don't burden yourself trying to do small group work in your bustling and harried public space. You will just be frustrated.

Mark 5:18-20 – What's *Your* Proclamation?

Some are called to be apostles, prophets, evangelists, or pastor-teachers. However, most people aren't. So what are they to proclaim in the public spaces? The same as the man healed of 2,000 demons. Tell others what the Lord has done for *you* and the loving mercy He has had on *you*. Proclaim what God has done for *you*, is doing for *you*, and/or has promised to do for *you* in challenging circumstances similar to what your peers or patients are going through. Tell a relevant story of *your* walk with Jesus. Who can argue? Lest you think this is not an effective strategy, read Mark 5:1-20 and then read Mark 6:53-56. Ask yourself, "What happened to the hearts and minds of the people of the region to make such a difference in their response to Jesus?"

Acts 1:8 – Receive God's Power to Proclaim *Your* Witness of Christ

What was the difference between the Peter who withered at the feet of a little girl when asked about Jesus and the bold Peter of Pentecost and Solomon's Colonnade? ONLY ONE THING: Peter had received the power of the indwelling Holy Spirit of God. Every believer is sealed and indwelled by the Holy Spirit. The promised power of God to be His witnesses is certainly available. But do you recognize and receive Him? Do you claim Him as the equipping gift from God the Father for you in your situation?

May these thoughts set you on the path to be joyous and free to do the good works God has prepared in advance for you to do.

⌒ Public-Space Proclamations

We have addressed in broad strokes some of the barriers, the "Yeah, buts...," that keep us from saying anything 'spiritual' to our peers or patients, even when we have a clear sense we ought to. One hindrance was the failure to recognize life is made up of public spaces where proclamations are made and private spaces for dialogue and discipleship (Acts 2:46-47). When we miss the distinction, we get frustrated about not having enough time or a good setting for 'spiritual talk' in our workplace. Relief from some of our frustration is found in acknowledging our public space and tailoring our respectful, sensitive, and appropriate spiritual statements to brief proclamations.

What is a Proclamation?

If we look at how Jesus used them, we might define a proclamation as *a brief statement that speaks truth and either explicitly or implicitly invites the hearer to reflect and respond toward that truth.*

In Scripture, we can see at least three ways God makes proclamations. The first way God made spiritual proclamations is through our environment – creation in some cases, situations in others. Psalm 19 and Romans 1, for example, describe this. Previously in these notes of encouragement, we have discussed the importance of proclaiming that we serve the God of peace, hope, and comfort by carefully creating a waiting area or practice space which fosters these things and invites people to open the door to their spiritual life.

> Proclamations don't have to be long-winded or preachy.

Secondly, in cases where a hearer came to Jesus intentionally to discuss spirituality, Jesus made His proclamation to the person directly. For example, in John 3, Jesus spoke in bold proclamations straight to Nicodemus. Jesus could do this forthrightly because Nicodemus had expressly asked Jesus about spiritual issues.

Third, in situations where Jesus had a proclamation for an audience that did not come to hear spiritual words, such as those who came for a meal or to be healed, Jesus often directed His proclamation elsewhere, knowing the intended audience could overhear it. This 'bank-shot' technique took many forms: praying out loud (speaking of or to Himself, so to speak), speaking to His disciples in the presence of a larger crowd, or addressing a single person's or group's erroneous teachings or inappropriate actions in the midst of a greater gathering. In our busy and crowded settings, this 'bank-shot' way of making a proclamation is very often an effective technique.

As we can see then, there are many ways we might make proclamations about God in our public space. Proclamations don't have to be long-winded or preachy. They can sow seeds, water, weed, or occasionally be an instrument used by the Master for harvesting. But if we do not ever make any proclamations, we will never sow, water, weed or harvest in our practice. Certainly that is not what we want.

In the next Note, we will take up the subject of *your* proclamation. Rooted in Mark 5:18-20, we will discover our proclamations are much more personal and relational than we might have thought possible. As such, they can bear a tremendous amount of fruit without being confrontational, offensive, or 'against the rules.'

☙ What's Your Proclamation?

Previously, we observed that in our busy settings we don't have time to be preachy or deeply theological. (Along with time crunches, there are obviously other reasons to consider whether that is even appropriate in a seven-minute visit.) However, we did note that there are good, biblical reasons to freely express a proclamation in such a public setting. We defined a proclamation as *a brief statement that speaks truth and either explicitly or implicitly invites the hearer to reflect and respond toward that truth.*

So the question becomes, "Proclaim what?" We also are led to wonder whether a short statement can have any real and lasting value, or whether, maybe, it just makes us feel good. To find the answers to those questions, I really urge you to take time to look at your favorite translation of two familiar passages from the Gospel of Mark: 4:35-5:20 and 6:45-56.

Bible Background

To be very succinct in looking at these passages side-by-side, here is a summary.

- Both stories feature physical storms on water – the 'as they went' storms.

- Both stories feature body, soul, and spirit storms on land – the 'where they live' storms.

- Both stories feature corporate storms – group troubles, even for Jesus' followers.

- Both stories feature private storms – troubles for individuals and families.

- Both stories begin on the Sea of Galilee and end on the far-east shore regions.

- Both stories feature Jesus as the penultimate healing, teaching, and preaching hero.

So why tell these two stories? If they are so similar, what critical lesson is the Holy Spirit trying to teach us that requires recounting these two events? It is the value of making a proclamation; a personal "this is my story with God" declaration.

In the first passage, there were numerous eyewitnesses to Jesus healing a man possessed of many demons (sick of soul), self-mutilating (sick of body), and starving for God to help him (sick of spirit). In other words, the whole person needed God and God came to save him wholly. But how did the witnesses react? Even though witnesses saw the healing event, they actually urged Jesus to leave.

In the second passage, when Jesus returned to the area, people came flooding to Him from everywhere, bringing themselves or their sick friends and loved ones. Jesus healed them all. What a dramatic change of heart the people of the region had, especially considering Jesus had left the region at their request!

What happened to make the difference in the hearts of the people? Why did the people turn towards Jesus rather than push Him away again?

KEY: It was the personal proclamation of the man whom Jesus had healed in the graveyard. Jesus told this fellow to go home to his family, his peeps, his posse, and tell *his* story of what the Lord had done for *him* and the loving mercy God had had on *him*. No mention of the Roman Road or The Four Spiritual Laws. No theology lessons or quoting endless

Scripture verses. Not even a call to repent. Just, 'Go tell *your* story of how God touched *you*.'

On his own initiative, the man told his story in ten cities. Unable to argue with the man about his own story, apparently his proclamations caused many people to reflect on what they had heard. They became willing to give Jesus a first or second look. They were willing to let God be a part of their own story of being wholly healed too.

Application

Every one of us, if we are Christians, has a story with God. Depending upon our individual circumstances, the length and texture of it is likely different. No surprise – it is *your* story, not somebody else's. It is not your parents' or your pastor's story, but *yours*. However, according to Jesus, every one of these stories ought to feature one or two things.

First, you might proclaim what the Lord has done for *you*. Not what He promised to do for someone else, but for *you*. By virtue of your role in healthcare, the patients, families, and peers you engage presume you are an intelligent person who carefully considers facts. So when you say the Lord has done something for *you*, that carries a great deal of weight.

> Every one of us, if we are Christians, has a story with God.

In general, these would be statements about how God has interacted with your temporal life. These proclamations are about how He has encouraged, taught, delivered, healed, or blessed you. These ought to have a freshness and currency about them, if you have a deliberate and ongoing fellowship with Him. Many times, you might comment on how a Bible passage which is fitting to the other person's concern has helped *you*.

163

Second, you might proclaim the loving mercy God has had on *you*. How has God touched *your* life to relieve you of guilt over the past, the fears of today, or hopelessness regarding tomorrow? Here, as it is appropriate, is where you might proclaim the glories of the person and work of Jesus on *your* behalf. You might mention the eternal joy and hope He has brought *you*, regardless of your temporal circumstances.

Conclusion

Ask God to bring to mind the things the Lord has done for you and the loving mercy He has had on you. Make it fresh, not an ancient, dusty, musty story you are unenthusiastic about. Throughout history individuals telling their story of life with God have changed whole lands. The invitation stands for you to continue this glorious story, right where you practice or study. Amen.

You Will Receive Power

Dynamite with a fuse unlit

is only potential power.

With the fuse lit

it is transformed into kinetic energy,

unleashing tremendous power.

In a previous note of encouragement, we saw the difference in the Apostle Peter's ability to proclaim the Gospel in power after he received the Holy Spirit. Here are three brief points to consider when you doubt you have the knowledge or ability to give *your* proclamation of what the Lord has done for *you* and/or the loving mercy He has had on *you*.

Point 1 – The Holy Spirit, Already Given to You, Is POWER to Witness

Every believer receives the Holy Spirit – God – to live in him or herself. It is good to remember that this is the same Spirit who overshadowed Mary in order to conceive the sinless Son of God and Son of man. The same powerful Spirit raised Jesus from the dead 33 years later. He is the same Spirit who overcame all of your doubts, fears, and arguments, and illuminated the Scriptures so they would become believable to you. By the Holy Spirit's power you were born again, raised from spiritual deadness to newness of life! With such power available to you, how can you rationally doubt God will empower you to do what He has called you to do?

Point 2 – We Must Take Possession of God's Promises

If you are looking for a single chapter in Scripture that just quakes with God's power, you are hard pressed to surpass Deuteronomy 11. Embedded at the heart of the chapter is a critical principle for God's people: God may make a promise but *you* have to step out in faith and take possession of it. You will possess only the land you set foot on.

Jesus said in Acts 1 that we would receive the Holy Spirit in order to empower us to be His witnesses. However, we must believe Him, acting on that belief by opening our mouth and sharing *our* witness story. Think of it this way: dynamite with a fuse unlit is only potential power; with the fuse lit it is transformed into kinetic energy unleashing tremendous power. Will you live by faith and step out? Will you light the fuse with faith?

Point 3 – Prepare to Be Reminded

In John 14, Jesus told His disciples that the Holy Spirit would remind us of all that Jesus had said. 'Remind' clearly implies that God expects we have been available and listening. We have heard something from God, storing it away in the armory of our mind so that the Holy Spirit could later go there to draw out the right sword for the right situation.

Do you spend time in God's Word? That's where we hear from Jesus and we hear about Jesus. In our devotional time we read of His person and works, we gain insight into how He affected people of the past, recall how He touched our lives, and see what He has promised to do in the future for others. If you want the Holy Spirit to remind you of what to say, be diligent to spend time in God's Word.

Summary

Through this series on overcoming, we have recognized many of us do not salt or light our encounters with our patients for a host of reasons. We called those the "Yeah, buts." We've also learned that many of our excuses evaporate if we just remember three simple principles of speaking about Christ in our healthcare ministry.

First, use proclamations – short statements of truth that invite others to reflect or engage – rather than giving long-winded theology lessons.

Second, *your* proclamation of truth should speak of what the Lord has done for *you* and / or the loving mercy He has had on *you*. That way, as our own Dr. Bill Bixler has taught us, we *expose* Jesus rather than *impose* Him.

Third, step out in faith that as you have listened to God in your Bible study time, the Holy Spirit will remind you of the right proclamation for the right situation. You will receive POWER to be bold!

To God be all the glory. Amen.

ELISHA

From a healthcare perspective,

few people's lives recorded in Scripture

have as much to teach us.

Have your Bible at your side

as you take up the lessons from this eight-part study of

God's prophet to those in healthcare.

❧ The Early Lessons

Elisha is a superb candidate as a prophetic role model for healthcare workers. His history is in 1 & 2 Kings, where – observed in total – you can see Elisha's healthcare ministry. The initial text for this study is 1 Kings 19:15-21. We begin our study by looking in detail for important foundational lessons from his early, pre-prophet life which have application to our lives as Christian healthcare students and practitioners. I pray you will discover that the entire bloom of Elisha's healthcare ministry can be seen in the bud of these few verses.

Dealing with Death (v.15-17)

All Christians, by virtue of our obligation to share our testimony and spread the Gospel, are involved in spiritual life and death issues. Yet some of us are called to deal directly with the life, decay, or death of body and/or soul. If you meditate on it, regardless of your specific role in Christian healthcare, you will find that you too have a life and death calling like Elisha.

No Solo Acts (v.18)

Your calling is unique to you, as the Lord chose you for your specific ministry. However, you are not the only one God called or will call. You are part of a body of people God calls. They too have a role that is essential, according to God. These other people are all around you. You are not – as Elijah mistakenly thought – alone. Elijah's fear and burnout might well have been ameliorated had he built relationships with others. This seems to be a lesson Elisha took to heart, as we shall see.

Elisha's Foundational Character is Revealed (v.19)

Elisha was called while he was working in another arena. He was working hard at being productive where he was; he wasn't called out of a recliner with a game controller firmly in his grasp.

- Bringing up the rear was Elisha's position when he received God's calling (as it was for Joseph in Egyptian prison, Moses in the Midian wilderness, David in the Judean pastures, Gideon in the winepress in Ophrah and Jesus in Nazareth). God wants us to notice that Elisha was bringing up the rear, and not in the lead. Academically or athletically many of us may have been at the head of our peers, but God called the one faithfully serving at the back of the line. Study hard and play hard…but is your heart, your spirit, willing to be last? Jesus spent *years* teaching that lesson to the apostles. It remains a hard lesson for us to learn.

- Today, whatever your position in the pecking order, do you seek God's best for the rest? Many of us now practice or study with others who serve in a 'lesser,' 'back of the line' or 'lower rung' role. Do you ask God to let you throw His mantle over these others so they might discover His big plan for them? (Here's a challenge: Ask God to show you how you can throw His mantle over the ones who quietly clean your workplace, classroom, and restroom. After all, Elijah threw God's mantle over a man who daily plowed through the dung of at least 24 oxen.)

A Person of Loving Gratitude (v.20)

Elisha didn't forget to express honoring, loving gratitude to the ones who helped get him to this place of God's calling. Elijah encouraged this attitude. How about you? Are you a loving, grateful person to those who have helped you?

171

Elisha's Training and Tools Are Implements of Worship and Service (v.21)

- The oxen and tack were Elisha's to do with as he chose. He chose these critical things to symbolize the tone of his entire ministry.

- Elisha didn't leave himself with provision to turn back from his calling if things got tough. Scripture is replete with similar instructions.

- Elisha dedicated whatever he had to the worship of God.

- Part of Elisha's worship of God throughout his ministry stems from his generosity to and celebration with those around him. Elisha lived the Law in his ministry by loving God and his neighbors.

I hope you find encouragement in the early life and calling of Elisha. May he be a model for you to emulate. In future notes, we'll see his whole life has much to teach those of us in healthcare.

✌ Life in the Shadows Has Value

Please read the biblical text for this note of encouragement: 1 Kings 19c-2 Kings 1:18.

Elisha didn't begin his ministry by stealing Elijah's blazing spotlight. Instead, Elisha served for some number of years in Elijah's shadow. That's where he learned what it meant to follow, to seek God, and to be a leader of men under God's authority.

There is no shame in serving those who have more notoriety.

- Joseph served in the shadow of Potiphar and Pharaoh.

- Joshua was in Moses' shadow for decades.

- Somebody rarely considered as a role model for faithful second fiddle was Silas in the New Testament. Too bad. He served with James at the Jerusalem Council, went on missions and to the Philippian jail alongside Paul, and wrote one of Peter's epistles to the church. We all benefit by studying his biography.

When a season comes to learn while serving, don't seek the spotlight. Instead, welcome the preparation time. There is very much to learn and be thankful for in clerkships, residency, and fellowships. God will raise up His humble servants in due time.

✑ From Shadow to Leading Light

Caution is in order when reading 2 Kings 2 and finding application to our healthcare ministry. If you read it hastily, Elisha will come across as precisely the worst kind of role model for us – curt, rude, standoffish, and vindictive. Yet everything we know of him before and after this chapter reveals he is just the opposite. So take the time to hear God's voice as you read the text.

Focus, Focus, Focus (v.1-8)

According to God's command, Elijah had thrown his prophetic mantle over Elisha. The Lord had, in effect, called Elisha to his ministry and he knew it. Now as his time in class, time in internship, time in residency, time in fellowship was coming to a close, Elisha would not be distracted. Repeatedly he had chances to quit, to stand down, to not finish well in his time of training. He also ran a gauntlet of chattering choruses singing the refrain of the obvious and the distracting. The distracters were not paying attention to the Spirit and spiritual things happening right in front of them. They wanted Elisha unfocused too.

Elisha would not be detoured. He refused to take his eyes off the spiritual meaning of the events happening around and within himself. He kept his focus on the fact God had called him, provided training, and now was about to release him to serve. Elisha demonstrated spiritual focus.

Do you have Elisha's focus? Will you make a point of training to perform your ministry skillfully, as an act of worship? (Psalm 33:3) When faced with impending change, great responsibilities, storms breaking around you, winds of opposition, and chatterers of little faith distracting you, will you, like Elisha and Jesus (Mark 4:35-41) declare, "Be silent! Be still! I am faithfully focused"?

Focus Rewarded with Responsibility and Gifting (v.9-13)

Elisha had been under Elijah's tutelage for several years. Elisha was facing a King Solomon moment when he could ask for anything and get it. For most mortals, like Gehazi, that would have meant seeking material blessing. But similar to Solomon asking the Lord for wisdom to lead well, Elisha asked for a double portion of the Spirit of God which empowered Elijah.

Elijah replied that this request was difficult. Why? Some suggest it was because Elijah knew it would mean a heavy burden of responsibility on Elisha. Others suggest that taking the double portion would represent Elisha becoming the leader of all the prophets; he would have to contend with doubters and pretenders to the position among other prophets, as well as having to lead a backslidden nation to follow Yahweh.

However, consider this. As God said in Zechariah 4:6, God's anointed do not operate by their own might or power but by God's Holy Spirit. And the Holy Spirit is not for Elijah or any other person to give away or sell. Elijah could pray for Elisha and encourage him to finish focused. It would have to be the God who called Elisha who would give him, and fill him with, His Spirit.

Are you praying for those with whom you train and work? Do you encourage them to keep a spiritual focus on God? Do you show them how vitally important being filled with God's Spirit will be to being everything God calls a Christian healthcare worker to be? Are you praying to be Spirit-filled as you minister?

175

Not Everyone Around You Will Have Your Spiritual Focus
(v.14-18)

The passing of the mantle didn't happen in secret. Elisha tested it and many people witnessed it. Elisha recognized the responsibility given to him was of God. The God of fiery horses and chariots would be the power behind what Elisha could do. Do you recognize that, too? If not, why not?

Many of the people around Elisha bowed down to him and gave him tacit authority over them, but soon returned to operating from the flesh and living in the past. They wanted Elijah back. They wanted to go snipe hunting. Elisha wasn't embarrassed that he had to tell them not to go. As a prophet he would have to tell many people what to do and not do. He was embarrassed at how quickly those who were also called prophets lost spiritual focus and turned back to a yearning for the past, looking for some other way then what the Spirit wanted for this season. They weren't seeing with spiritual eyes.

As a Christian in healthcare, you recognize that the human beings coming to you are more than broken bodies or disturbed souls. They are spiritual creatures, too. You will again and again run into people who will give that idea lip service. They may challenge you when you try to integrate the spiritual into caring for your patients. Like Elisha, be embarrassed for them and have compassion. They don't know better . . . until you teach them.

The Salty Healer (v.19-22)

Related to this passage, two things are critical. First, Elisha gave the Lord credit for the healing of the water, transforming it from death to life. Elisha was called upon to effect a cure to a serious problem, but Elisha gave God the glory. Second, Jesus called us to be salty. In your practice, you are the bowl of salt. Your faith – which God has given you and called you to share through your witness – has a very definite place in effecting healing now and for eternity.

Dealing with the Devil (v.23-25)

Based upon how Elisha would soon deal with Gehazi's error, if the boys were merely making fun of Elisha's physical feature, Elisha might have simply made 42 bald little boys. Instead, he cursed them and turned them over to God for His judgment. This suggests that, lost to time's mists, the taunting was a manifestation of spiritual warfare. Once Elisha turned them over, he made a pilgrimage to Mt. Carmel, where his mentor Elijah was an instrument of God in one of the greatest spiritual battles ever recorded. Only after Elisha spent time in such a holy place did Elisha really begin his ministry.

Don't ever forget Christians in healthcare are engaged in spiritual battles. Sickness and death of the body, corruptions of the soul, and being born without a spirit connected to God are all the result of the Devil's temptations and Adam's succumbing. Some of these terrible evils today are made even worse by ongoing temptations, succumbing, and possibly even demonic oppression. Lest you think this is stretching the scope of your Christian healthcare ministry, recall what the Apostle Paul says:

> *Don't ever forget Christians in healthcare are engaged in spiritual battles.*

> *For our battle is not against flesh and blood, but against the rulers, against the authorities, against the world powers of this darkness, against the spiritual forces of evil in the heavens. This is why you must take up the full armor of God, so that you may be able to resist in the evil day, and having prepared everything, to take your stand. …With*

177

every prayer and request, pray at all times in the
Spirit, and stay alert in this, with all perseverance
and intercession for all the saints.

Ephesians 6:12-14, 18

May God give us the Elisha-like focus to finish our tasks faithfully. May we be faithful to give God glory, seek the Holy Spirit's help to care for people, stand on behalf of others against the Devil's schemes, and above all pray with compassion for one another as co-laborers in Christian healthcare ministry. May the Lord of fiery horses and chariots fill you to overflow with His Spirit.

⌒ Corruption & Compassion

The biblical text for this note of encouragement is 1 Kings 3.

Elisha finds himself a servant of God called to ministry at the behest of government agents. The godly king of Judah whom Elisha respects, in trying to make peace, allies himself with the wicked king of Israel, whom Elisha despises and disdains. A third king from Edom is a vassal king of the other two. The mixed bag of armies under these three kings are on the way to attack the nation of Moab, who was in rebellion against Israel.

After a week of marching, the combined armies find themselves in dire straits before ever engaging Moab. They are without water for man or military beast. So they call upon Elisha for aid and counsel. What did Elisha do? What lessons can we learn from his actions? And what can we learn about our God as well?

Elisha makes clear his preferred king is the godly one. He does not refrain from honestly expressing face-to-face his disdain for another ruler because that one openly opposes God and is an oppressor of people. Elisha recognizes his primary responsibility and service is to God, before government. Yet as a citizen, he knows he is also responsible to those in authority over him. Therefore, rather than acting from his preference or his flesh, he seeks God's instruction for how to proceed.

(How cool was it that Elisha seemed to need background music to hear from God? See Psalm 33:3, Ephesians 5:19-21, and Colossians 3:16-17.)

Elisha, at the direction of God, gives guidance which will preserve the life of the men and beasts before him. Though

179

there were unpleasant features about Elisha's situation, he understood at that time and place, God's use of his ministry was to meet the physical needs of those looking to him for help in their time of life-threatening danger.

Elisha's ministry was *also* to speak God's Word to the leaders; not just meet physical needs, but speak God's plan into their lives. But what about the fact that these men were saved to go make war on Moab? That was not, at that time and place (as it would be at the end of Elisha's life) his concern or responsibility. Elisha accepted that God had control of the situation and final outcome.

At the sight of a blazing human sacrifice on a Moabite city wall, great sickness and wrath came upon the Israelite army. Even after all the lives lost and destruction caused, Israel's wicked king returned home having not accomplished the oppressive goal for which he set out.

Applications

Do you recognize that God is ultimately in charge of your healthcare ministry? One evidence of whether you *really* believe that is that you pray for Him to guide your interactions with your patients, peers, and authorities.

In the face of unpleasant situations and bureaucratic mandates, do you strive to keep your focus on the patients and their needs? You can't fix the world, but you can be God's agent of grace in solving the problems right before you.

Do you make a habit of not only meeting physical needs, but listening to God and speaking His Truth into your patients' lives as well? If not, why not?

❧ Soul-Care & the Widow's Oil

In this note of encouragement, we see the beginning of Elisha's healthcare ministry. His first act is not a physical healing, but a process of soul-care. Why should most of us be interested? Because Christians in healthcare follow in the footsteps of Jesus, not only healing bodies, but teaching people's souls (emotions, intellect, memories, and will) and speaking to their spirits. The Bible text is 2 Kings 4:1-7.

Elisha's 'Patient': A Very Volatile Situation (v.1)

The first thing we should observe is the tremendous stress this poor woman is under. All at once, she presents to Elisha crying out in anguish. She has the grief of her husband's death. She has two sons to take care of – they are not old enough to take care of her. She fears for their lives in impending slavery, plus what that will mean for her future as well. Her family is disintegrating before her eyes. She appears to be isolated, not having any other family from which to get help. Her finances are a wreck. Who among us would not hurt for her if she appeared before us?

**Elisha's Godly Character and Wisdom
Help Establish an Initial Plan** (v.2-5)

We've previously noted how Elisha cares for the people around him. He has compassion on their plights. He loves his neighbors. As a Christian serving through healthcare, you do too, even if you are not a prophet.

Elisha asked questions and let the woman give answers before anything else. He helped her prioritize what mattered most. Then he explored her resources with her. He wasn't thinking about how to 'fix' her problem at the outset. He was helping *her* process options and evaluate *her* resources.

Now comes that part which is unique to us as Christians – our access to the Godly wisdom Elisha had. Elisha had a double portion of God's Spirit *on* him; you have the Holy Spirit *in* you. He knows what you need before you ask, because He communes with your spirit, He prays on your behalf when you don't know what to pray, He reminds you of the things Jesus taught, the One who is wisdom personified, and as James 1:5-8 says, He will give you the wisdom you need if you will believe and decisively obey what He tells you.

> Our task is to be so in tune with God through faith, Bible study, and prayer, that we can confidently point those who are in need of soul-care to the One who can meet every need.

Elisha gave the woman a simple, clear, manageable pair of action steps: borrow all the pots you can and fill them. Yes, God was going to do a miracle. But what you need also to see is that Elisha didn't feel a burden to solve her problem out of *his* resources. He tested the widow to see if she would let God help her. Too many of us doubt God will help, so we don't send our patients to seek God's help either. That certainly isn't what we see in Elisha's ministry.

The Widow's Part (v.5b-6)

The woman did everything she was told. Only then did she come back to Elisha.

Elisha's Concluding Counsel (v.7)

Elisha's counsel (which he had time to think about in the meantime, before the 'next appointment'), continued to point her to God's faithfulness to care for her and her sons – the widow and orphans God cares about so much. The God of the birds and the lilies would attend to her immediate and long term needs. He knows them all. He cares. Elisha's final counsel was specific – go, sell, pay off, live. But more importantly, it offered her hope through the work of God in her life, now and always.

Application

Elisha loved his neighbors (the ones at hand whom he could help) and thus demonstrated his love for God. He lived the royal law. Sometimes, as in the feeding of the 4,000 and 5,000 with a few fish and loaves, God will test you by asking you to reach into your resources, or those you have access to. However, more often than not, our task is to be so in tune with God through faith, Bible study, and prayer, that we can confidently point those who are in need of soul-care to the One who can meet every need.

Do you trust God? Do you encourage your patients to put their trust in Him also? Do you go with them to God's throne in prayer and ask Him to help the helpless?

↷ The Big Itch Named Isolation

These lessons don't come out of a vacuum but out of *your* real life stories. In meeting with folks all over North Carolina, one story replays over and over. I call it the "big itch of isolation." This itch needs a good scratch!

As Christians, you have probably noticed Solomon's admonition to have one or two relationships upon which you can rely (Ecclesiastes 4:9-12). Or that Jesus almost invariably sent His followers out into the world in pairs or triplets. Or that the apostles followed Jesus' model by almost always ministering in the company of fellow believers. Jesus promised that where two or more gathered to pray in His name, He would be with them (Matthew 18:19-20).

> We need a ministry partner with whom we can talk and share our struggles.

Yet for a host of reasons, too many healthcare students and practitioners allow themselves to practice in a state of soul isolation. They don't have one or two fellow students or practitioners with whom they join for mutual soul-care.

Isolation was an error Elisha learned to guard against through hearing of his mentor Elijah's 'Woe is me' despair in a cave (1 Kings 19:1-18). God is with us (His indwelling Spirit can't get any closer), yet even the powerful prophet Elijah's behavior demonstrated that broken people like ourselves need the soul-care and encouragement of a fellow believer we can see and touch. So let's look at an example of how avoiding isolation turned into soul-care in Elisha's ministry and find some application for ourselves. The Bible text is 2 Kings 4:8-37.

184

A Divine Appointment: Trust God to Introduce (v.8-10)

We have no information on how God orchestrated Elisha (and his ministry partner Gehazi) being invited to dinner by the Shunammite woman and her husband. What we do know is that over time, all four developed a strong relationship. The woman, through that relationship, recognized Elisha had a soul need – a place of quiet refuge and rest, and an assurance Gehazi's physical requirements would be met as well. So she joined with her husband to make provision to meet Elisha's needs and care for his soul.

Soul-Care May Take Time and Trust in God (v.11-17)

It took time and perception on Elisha's and Gehazi's part to discern the Shunammite's heartache and determine what her soul-need was. It also took a strong relationship with God not to make a rash statement regarding the fulfillment of her need. The key points of this section are that there was the commitment of meeting together to have the relationship, and there was a deep trust in God to help identify and address the Shunammite's real issue.

**Testing Your Commitment to Each Other –
Be Faithful, Not Fickle** (v.18-37)

When the storm comes to your friend – night falls, winds howl, breaking waves crash over the gunnels – will you be found faithful to the fellowship God has fostered, or will you be AWOL? This story isn't suggesting that you somehow adopt your fellowship partner, with all the responsibilities that come with adoption. God has already adopted him and will take that responsibility. However, you may be His instrument for his soul-care in a crisis. Moses needed Aaron and Hur at his side in a battle (Exodus 17:8-13), Jesus needed the Three Amigos in Gethsemane (Matthew 26:36-46), and the Shunammite woman needed Elisha.

185

When your fellowship partner needs soul-care in a crunch situation, will you be found faithful to make time for her or him? After all, that's no more or less then doing for others as you would want them to do for you (Matthew 7:12).

Application

Nobody is going to understand grief over loss or error, time pressures, financial concerns, family tribulations, or burn-out in healthcare like another person who is in a healthcare setting similar to yours. They may or may not be in your office. You might have to do as Elisha did and make deliberate plans to travel to the Shunammite's. However, this is an effort worth the small cost. We need a ministry partner with whom we can talk and share our struggles. Study and/or practice in isolation is, for every Christian, setting ourselves up as easy prey for the roaring lion seeking a saint (and thus a Christian medical ministry) to devour.

> *Be sober! Be on the alert! Your adversary the Devil is prowling around like a roaring lion, looking for anyone he can devour. Resist him, firm in the faith, knowing that the same sufferings are being experienced by your brothers in the world.*
>
> 1 Peter 5:8-9

∂ᴓ We All Serve God

Our text is 2 Kings 5:1-19, the account of the healing of Naaman the leper. This is one of those passages in Scripture with which I fear many of us have become too familiar, meaning we think we know what's there. So please, if you are able, read the text again with an open mind to see some things new and applicable to you.

Just because he was different didn't mean God didn't have a plan for Naaman, too (v.1)

No doubt Naaman was a warrior held in great esteem by the king of Aram, Israel's enemy. So our first reaction to him might be like that of Jonah to the Ninevites – 'Hate 'em all!' But God was using Naaman. Naaman had value to God. We need to guard against any personal preferences or prejudices blinding us to the value of all people to God. As followers of Jesus, all people should be valuable to us as well.

The least of these may be the lynchpin to complete healing (v.2-4)

God has a penchant for the small things and the 'little' people. Such terms are value judgments people make, often in error. Just pause for 30 seconds and recount how many youngsters and slaves God used to do His bidding in revealing hearts or changing nations. Christian receptionists, billers, CNAs, etc. all can – and do – have the potential to join with you in being agents of God's grace and healing. Often they will see or hear things from patients they might not say to you, or express an emotion after they

> Healthcare is a complex undertaking, involving many team members.

187

have left you that signals there is a need for acute body, soul, and spiritual care of which you were unaware. Don't discount their importance to God's work and your healthcare ministry.

Be aware of the larger audience (v.5-7)

Suffice it to say there is often an audience to your care for a patient. They may not understand what is happening any better than the patient. This sets up the potential for conflict. It also presents an opportunity for teaching and spreading grace. Don't ignore the bystanders.

Yes, the patient came to see you, but will they see God, too? (v.8-12)

Let's get the obvious out of the way first: you must be the very best healthcare provider you can be. That goes without saying. So you can't sit behind a green curtain and send out orders via a messenger without seeing the patient. Duh.

Now look deeper.

Elisha's tactic was not to be coy, but to get Naaman to focus on YHWH, the God of Israel, not on Elisha the man. Elisha had a goal for Naaman to be healed of skin disease, but he had an even higher goal of leading Naaman to know the One who had orchestrated his life and had plans for him. Naaman's anger wasn't so much that he didn't get to see Elisha as it was that Naaman had certain plans for how things were supposed to happen and God, through Elisha, ordered Naaman's steps down a completely different path (see Proverbs 16:9). Wrapped up in this passage is the whole humanity of Naaman – body, soul, and spirit – and the holistic care God and Elisha had for Naaman.

Do you look at and care for your patients and peers holistically? If not, why not? God does.

Serving a prodigal commander in a far country (v.13-14)

Again, the 'little people' are used by God to dispense wisdom. We wonder whether Naaman, if he was back home in Damascus, would have given them the time of day, let alone listen to their counsel? There is also the issue of having to travel to a far land to hear God's voice. Whether the patient in front of you comes from a background of privilege or prosperity, or has lived a life of dissipation, are you sensitive to the fact that the troubles of their body or soul have led them to you, in a far land they never planned to visit? Will you listen to and be the voice of the Holy Spirit if He prompts you to speak of God as the eternal healer and ever-present comfort in times of trouble?

Elisha, like Jesus, saw physical or soul healing as a platform for promoting the spirit's health (v.15-16)

Elisha never asked Naaman, "How's that skin thing?" or "Got control of your anger problem, yet?" Instead, he heard God working in the spiritual life of Naaman and made a point of shunning anything that would impede God's work there. When the Holy Spirit is moving to bring a person to eternal life, strive to keep the patient and their audience focused upon and listening to Him.

"Go in peace" (v.17-19)

What a statement for all of us to adopt! He who began a good work in Naaman would be faithful to complete it. What an encouraging thing to know and to share with our patients. We don't have to shepherd them through seminary. We just need to remind them to trust God to continue to work in their lives, if they will set their mind to follow Him. As God ordered Naaman's circumstances to get him to Elisha's clinic and home again, so we can trust Him to shepherd our patient when he leaves.

189

Application

This historic account is replete with characters great and small. Each had a role. The key to Naaman's complete healing was that everyone did their part. Healthcare is a complex undertaking, involving many team members. Do you foster a sense of ministry responsibility among all your Christian circle? Do you appreciate the role each person fulfills? Are you fulfilling your Christian calling to see every person as valuable and caring for them holistically, as God leads and presents opportunities?

᧤ Discipling Through Mistakes

Have you ever made a mistake? I mean a really big one. I have. Once, in haste, I gave the wrong drug to a patient. I could have killed her; blessedly there was actually no adverse outcome. Since I was alone and there was no apparent harm, I could have hidden the error and nobody would have been any the wiser. But I chose to self-report. I was first met with amazement. Then I received graceful, merciful mentoring. The event will forever be a defining component of who I am and how I relate to others.

Lurking in the shadows of Elisha's story as the healthcare prophet has been this fellow named Gehazi. He really blew it too. Then he also tried to hide his poor choice – his sinful faithlessness in God. How Elisha related to Gehazi has much to show those of us who, by either our position or vocation, are mentors to others in healthcare.

> Do we define people by occasional errors or by their life's trajectory?

How should we respond to those around us who make a mistake or a bad choice? Does how we deal with them depend upon the event or how our 'disciple' responds to the event? Do we define people by occasional errors or by their life's trajectory? Elisha's model helps us answer these questions. Our texts are excerpts from 2 Kings 4-8.

Gehazi was Elisha's Disciple (4:12, 5:20, 8:4)

Elisha had a cadre of students serving around and with him, called the 'sons of the prophets.' Yet repeatedly in our texts, Gehazi is recognized as someone very close to Elisha – his attendant or servant. It seems everywhere Elisha went, there was Gehazi. Whether explicitly or implicitly, Gehazi was a disciple of Elisha. Elisha, as evidenced by the overall story, certainly took an interest in teaching Gehazi about living and working by faith.

Do you have one or more disciples? Especially in the high pressure, privileged role as a Christian in healthcare you should. You should have a mentor, too. Who teaches you how to be an excellent student or practitioner *and* an excellent Christ follower? Who are you teaching to integrate faith in God with care for the body, soul and spirit of patients?

Blowing It Big Time: The End for Gehazi? (chapter 5)

Gehazi had seen Elisha raise the dead, cleanse a poisoned stew, and feed 100 grown men with just 20 barley buns. Gehazi should have been able to walk by faith in God. Yet the evidence of the kinds of things Gehazi did showed that his faith in God's plan and provision for him was weak. God allows us to be tested, not so He can figure out who we are – He certainly already knows – but so *we* can learn who we are. And so those around us can know too.

Who gave Gehazi leprosy? Don't forget that the spirit that saw Gehazi (5:26) was most likely Elisha's double portion of the Holy Spirit (2 Kings 2:9-15). The spirit of Elisha to be a prophet was God's Spirit. Gehazi's faithlessness, deceitful acquisition of booty, and lying about it all may have hurt Elisha's feelings and trust, but they were an affront to God's reputation and plan. Elisha the prophet didn't give Gehazi leprosy. God, in His authority, did.

Elisha had to make an important choice. Would he define Gehazi forever as 'unclean,' a sinner, and cast him away? Or would Elisha show the redemptive character of Christ? Elisha could not change the consequence of Gehazi's sin, but he could act like Christ toward him, with merciful grace.

Elisha Asks God to Buttress Gehazi's Faith –
God of Second Chances (6:8-17)

Fondly, we may wish we could have something similar happen for us. Let's look critically though. First, we are called to walk by faith, not by sight. Second, Elisha had to pray for this because he was trying to redeem the faith of Gehazi, a faith that should have been strong enough to trust God.

However, let's also praise God He answered Elisha's prayer because He is a God of redemption. Let's also recognize that Elisha still had Gehazi at his side, despite his past failures, and was trying to build him up in his faith.

How are you at looking at the person working or studying alongside you? Do you see them as God does, as worthy of redemption, if they are repentant? Surely some of you may be thinking this sort of challenge is 'too theological' and has little to do with healthcare. But isn't your faith in the Gospel supposed to change you entirely into a new creation, one moving towards fulfilling God's image and likeness in the world, and expressing that in the good works *God* has prepared for you to do? If that faith is alive in you, then your deeds toward others in need of redeeming grace in your classroom or practice should reflect that, shouldn't it?

Demonstrating Gehazi's Growth (8:16)

What fruits do we see in Gehazi in this vignette? First, Gehazi is looking back on a faith event with fondness and enthusiasm. Second, Gehazi was there at the raising of the dead son too. Yet his focus is on his master's model of faith in God and the work it wrought. Third, Gehazi's error was the injustice of accumulating material goods for himself at the cost of God's reputation. Now, however, we see Gehazi striving as God's agent of grace to use his situation to see that the Shunammite woman receives justice and has her possessions returned. What a marvelous turnaround!

Applications

Lesson 1. We have very serious responsibilities in health-care, and even more so as Christians, for the quality of our work unto the Lord is in many ways reflected in the caliber of the care we give our patients. Sins repented of are forgiven, but by virtue of the fact they are sins, they still have consequences. So do medical errors. That necessarily being said, does Jesus define *you* by *your* mistakes? Doesn't He say, "Neither do I condemn you. Go and sin no more."? Do we at least consider that stance in our discipling roles at work or school?

Lesson 2. We all are subject to authorities in our practices. There are standardized expectations and consequences for violating the standards. If we fail to recognize that, we err. However, we can act mercifully and redemptively toward those who make a mistake or sin. We can do unto others as we would have them do to us. We can maintain high standards and still be agents of grace. We have great sway over how a person is defined into their future – by their error or their trajectory. How will we use that sway? Hopefully like the maturing Gehazi, Elisha's disciple.

PRACTICE TIPS

See one, do one, teach one.

That's a familiar medical adage.

It undergirds our studies, clerkships,

residencies, and fellowships.

The same adage applies to practicing Christian healthcare.

Here's a closing collection of procedures

to see, do, and teach.

❧ Lemonade Out of Lemons

Electronic medical records (EMR) have become the bane and number one complaint of Christians in healthcare. And not just Christians. EMR has been the subject of scathing commentaries in secular media and has been cited as a major contributing factor in the rise of practitioner burnout. In addition, patients feel neglected by the time practitioners now devote to computers. The care and feeding of a database has trumped patient care, despite what promoters say.

EMRs are here to stay, though. So Christians need to study God's playbook on how to handle adversity. Whether it's Joseph's attitude found in Genesis 50:20, or the Apostle Paul's reassurance found in Romans 8:28, Scripture tells us that God can make something good come from adversity. He creates lemonade out of lemons. We should learn to take the sour fruit of EMR and parlay it into an opportunity to refresh as well. Here are some ways.

> Christians need to study God's playbook on how to handle adversity.

While entering your patient's name, you can mention you find encouragement in Isaiah 49:16 which says the names of God's beloved people are written in the palms of His hands. God knows our names. Being all-knowing, He doesn't need a computer!

Inputting the patient's complaint, remark how when you feel burdened, you read Matthew 11:28-30 where Jesus invites everyone who is weary and burdened to come to Him for rest. He's all-powerful and wants to share our load.

As you type the treatment plan, you can reference Jeremiah 29:11-13, where God says He already has a plan for each of us. He's concerned for our well-being. He wants us to have hope. He desires we have a future with Him. Proclaim how you find that very uplifting.

These are just a few examples of how Christian healthcare is distinctive. We find ways to expose, not impose, Jesus. We offer spiritual hope. We work with the Holy Spirit and God's Word to redeem that which seems broken – even EMR. Practicing Christian healthcare can even turn our laptop into a lemonade stand of refreshing!

❧ Have You Found a Spiritual Voice?

In places like the Duke Physician Assistant school or the UNC Pharmacy school, Christians meet weekly to find out how to apply the Scriptures to the practice of Christian healthcare. Going through the Gospel of Mark, verse by verse, we discover that Christian healthcare isn't a matter of being the nicest, most compassionate, or most competent caregiver. Lots of faiths (and even atheists) encourage compassionate and competent care. Providing Christian healthcare is so much deeper and richly detailed than that.

We are discovering together that a distinctive mark of Christian healthcare is that practitioners find and use their 'spiritual voice.' Jesus spoke God's plan for humanity's redemption. He gave that calling to His followers. Christ followers, wherever they work, are to be God's redemptive messengers to the whole world (see 2 Corinthians 5:14-6:2).

I thought you might like to get a sample of how that message is communicated throughout the Gospel of Mark. This is a great example of how studying the person and work of Jesus through the gospels can and should shape how we view our full-orbed Christian practice of medicine. (Note: Don't be put off by the use of the word 'preach.' One could just as well use the words speak, proclaim, tell, or share.)

> *So He (Jesus) went into all of Galilee, preaching in their synagogues and driving out demons.*
>
> Mark 1:39

> *He also appointed 12 – He also named them apostles – to be with Him, to send them out to preach.*
>
> Mark 3:14

But He would not let him, (the demon-delivered man who wanted to go with Jesus), *"Go back home to your own people, and report to them how much the Lord has done for you and how He has had* (loving) *mercy on you." So he went out and began to proclaim in the Decapolis how much Jesus had done for him, and they were all amazed.*

Mark 5:19-20

So they (the apostles) *went out and preached that people should repent.*

Mark 6:12

Then He (Jesus) *said to them, "Go into all the world and preach the gospel to the whole creation.*

Mark 16:15

And they went out and preached everywhere, the Lord working with them and confirming the word by the accompanying signs.

Mark 16:20

The whole world, metaphorically, is coming to see you. With gentleness, respect, discernment, and also with Holy Spirit-provided power and boldness (Acts 1:8), have you found your spiritual voice and made it a part of how you provide true Christian healthcare ... healthcare that can last for an eternity? Do you pray for or with those to whom you minister through healthcare? Do you expose Jesus (not impose Him) by sharing what the Lord has done for *you* and the loving mercy He's had on *you*? That's using your spiritual voice to bring salt and light to your patient and peer encounters.

199

❧ Spiritual Vision

As Christians in healthcare, we have that privileged position of walking right in the footsteps of Jesus and the disciples. Like them, we often have the opportunity to heal bodies, teach souls, and speak to spirits all in a single encounter. But the disciples didn't learn how to do it overnight. It took time and training, just as it does for us. That includes learning how to have spiritual vision; seeing our patients, peers, and ourselves as God does.

Mark 8 is all about gaining spiritual vision. It is hard work to learn this lesson. Teaching it was frustrating for the Lord Himself. We observe Jesus:

- sighed deeply in consternation when religious rulers didn't see what God sees;

- asked tough, sardonic questions when disciples didn't see as God saw;

- spit in the eyes of a man gone blind from Bethsaida, a village that wouldn't see God's signs and which fell under God's wrath; and,

- threatened God's shame upon those who will not see with His eternal perspective on life.

Given these multiple examples of Jesus' frustration over spiritual blindness, it is reasonable to presume we need to sharpen our spiritual vision, if we are going to follow and serve Him in our healthcare ministry. We need to focus on those who have come to us for help, using God's eyes as well as our own.

Fortunately, Mark's gospel features more than Jesus' aggravation at spiritual blindness. The account also shows that those who are willing to see Jesus for who He is, are blessed. It demonstrates how even a person who comes from a despised town, and who *may* have gone blind as a result of his sin, can be healed.

How is your spiritual vision? Are you asking the Father to give you His insight every day for your situation and surroundings? Are you looking at your patients and peers in a loving, honest way, as God does? Only if you are exercising your spiritual vision can you truly walk in Jesus' footsteps in your healthcare ministry.

May you have eyes to see your patients and peers as God would have you truly to see them.

✑ He's Big Enough for Big Questions

In healthcare, we are constantly confronted with questions. The source for these questions is the soul – that immaterial, intangible place where our emotions, intellect, memories, and will come into confluence. No matter when, where, or how souls form, they all ask big questions and look for big answers. Since we are confronted with big questions, we think we have to have big answers. When we don't have them, we feel small and inadequate.

The brief book of Habakkuk is the account of a man asking big questions of God. When God answers his first questions, the answers seem so unfair that Habakkuk protests. In time, with gentleness, respect, and assurance, God responds to Habakkuk with more detail and clarity. Habakkuk still isn't convinced that what God is about to do is the right thing. That's actually okay with God, because God isn't looking to justify Himself or get a stamp of approval on His plans. What God sought and got from Habakkuk was an increase in, and expression of, faith that God's thoughts and ways, though higher and loftier than man's, can be trusted to be right.

> Since we are confronted with big questions, we think we have to have big answers. When we don't have them, we feel small and inadequate.

So what can we, as Christians in healthcare, learn from Habakkuk and God?

First, God is up to answering the really big questions. He's not offended if they are hard or challenge His fairness. So we shouldn't be afraid or offended when our patients ask the big questions.

Second, God doesn't expect we will understand everything He's doing. So the pressure is off us to explain Him or justify Him to others.

Third, what God really seeks is that people know Him. In that knowledge we discover He is loving, trustworthy, and will ultimately always be found to be just (fair, if you'd like).

That's the tack to take when helping your patients wrestle with the imponderables. Hopefully you will, with gentleness and respect, tell a bit of your story of how you've discovered God's loving, trustworthy character.

⤴ Who Are You Bringing Along?

> *Then the king promoted Daniel and gave him*
> *many generous gifts. He made him ruler over the*
> *entire province of Babylon and chief governor over*
> *all the wise men of Babylon. At Daniel's request,*
> *the king appointed Shadrach, Meshach, and Abed-*
> *nego to manage the province of Babylon. But Dan-*
> *iel remained at the king's court.*
>
> Daniel 2:48-49

Daniel and the boys were all taken captive together. They committed themselves to following God's Law together. They studied together. They proved themselves ten times wiser than all the other advisers in Nebuchadnezzar's kingdom together. For some reason, God chose to give the gift of knowing and interpreting dreams to Daniel. Yet even then, the trio faithfully prayed for Daniel to have the ability to use his gift and save innumerable lives. In short, God gives gifts, but faithfulness is demonstrated in both using those gifts for God's glory and not being puffed up by them.

> To be good is noble;
> but to show others
> how to be good
> is nobler
> and no trouble.
>
> Mark Twain

So when the king praised and elevated Daniel, Daniel not only gave God credit for his interpretive ability, but he asked the king to elevate his compadres too. Daniel didn't leave his faithful brothers behind to languish as just three among many in the king's court.

God has given us innate talents (1 Corinthians 4:7) and spiritual gifts as He saw fit (Ephesians 4:7, 11-13). Recognizing that, we are right to be wary of getting puffed up about our successes. We do well to remain humble and let God handle elevating us before men.

We also do well to remember those who have walked alongside us, prayed for us, and helped us get to where we are. Who among your circle of peers has stood with you, supported you, taught you and/or prayed for you? Are you, like Daniel, using your new-found position and influence to bring them along as well? Are you being a blessing to them as they have been to you?

❧ Do You Bring Good News?

Each of the synoptic Gospels reveals the same critical point about the ministry of Jesus and His followers: they preached the good news of God.

> *After John was arrested, Jesus went to Galilee, preaching the good news of God: "The time is fulfilled, and the kingdom of God has come near. Repent and believe in the good news!"*
>
> Mark 1:14-15

> *Every day in the temple complex and in various homes, they* (the apostles) *continued teaching and proclaiming the good news that Jesus is the Messiah. ...So those who were scattered* (non-apostolic followers) *went on their way preaching the message of good news.*
>
> Acts 5:42, 8:4

Very often this proclaiming of the good news was in conjunction with healing (Luke 9:6).

It is in the nature of medicine that we are news bearers. Not all news we bring is good news, as far as this mortal life goes. But as Christian healthcare practitioners, walking as the apostles and early disciples did in the footsteps of Jesus' healing, teaching and preaching, we should always have good news to share with every person. Obviously it requires discernment as to how and when to share it. But the news that God loves all people – wants to see all people live eternally in His glorious presence and love – remains good news of great joy for all people (Luke 2:8-14).

When you enter the presence of your patients, do you do so knowing that God has given you the role and opportunity to be a good news bearer? Do you pray daily asking the Holy Spirit to give you discernment to recognize your divine opportunity each day to proclaim that good news with joy and boldness? If not, why not? It is your divine assignment (2 Corinthians 5:16-21). Be a bearer of God's good news every day.

The angel said to them, "Don't be afraid,

for look, I proclaim to you good news of

great joy that will be for all the people.

Today a Savior, who is Messiah the Lord,

was born for you in the city of David.

Luke 2:10-11

☙ Words of Comfort

> *Praise the God and Father of our Lord Jesus Christ, the Father of mercies and the God of all comfort. He comforts us in all our affliction, so that we may be able to comfort those who are in any kind of affliction, through the comfort we ourselves receive from God. For as the sufferings of Christ overflow to us, so through Christ our comfort also overflows.*
>
> 2 Corinthians 1:3-5

Often I visit Christians in healthcare who, like Christ, have a real heart and compassion for those who hurt. However, they are not sure what to say to or how to pray with their patients who are afflicted, brokenhearted, crushed, or wounded. So they say nothing. Here are helpful ideas for speaking comfort.

Recognize you are God's ambassador of comfort. Your assignment is to share the comfort you have received. Since that is true, then it follows the God who appointed you ambassador and indwells you with the resurrection power of the Holy Spirit will give you the words, if you will ask Him.

You don't have to know every detail of what is going on in the mind of your patient. That's God's job. We comfort with the comfort we have received. Ask yourself, "If I were in my patient's situation, what comfort would I want from God?" Then pray for that with conviction for your patient.

Admit it. Some aspects of your patient's situation are beyond your skills or resources to fix. But you know the One who knows and can do all. Point your patient

> Recognize you are God's ambassador of comfort.

to Him. These two verses are a perfect and peace-bringing way to do that: *The LORD is near the brokenhearted; He saves those crushed in spirit. ...He heals the brokenhearted and binds up their wounds* (Psalm 34:18 & 147:3, see also Isaiah 61:1-2 & Luke 4:18, pointing to Jesus as this Great Physician).

You are an excellent practitioner as well as a trusted and faithful ambassador of God's grace. You can speak and pray His words of comfort. It's your privilege.

ϖ Our Ministry to Teach Souls

In her story, "Traps," Dr. Rachel Naomi Remen recounts a patient who, over the course of many years of struggling with heart disease, noted that increases in her angina pain correlated with bouts of self-deception. Her heart pain signaled soul trouble. After restorative surgery, the patient realized the gift of pain leading to self-discovery had left her. Only in hindsight did the patient and her doctor recognize the stone the builder's rejected had become a cornerstone of life (Rachel Naomi Remen, MD, *Kitchen Table Wisdom*, New York, Riverhead Books, 1996, pp. 75-77).

The concept of the rejected stone becoming the cornerstone first appears as part of a larger passage found in Psalm 118.

> *I will give thanks to You because You*
> *have answered me and have become my salvation.*
> *The stone that the builders rejected*
> *has become the cornerstone.*
> *This came from the LORD;*
> *it is wonderful in our eyes.*
> *This is the day the LORD has made;*
> *let us rejoice and be glad in it.*
>
> Psalm 118:21-24

What a profound declaration. So much so, Jesus is quoted using verse 118:22 in all three synoptic gospels and Peter used it in his apologetic (Acts 4:11), and again in his first epistle (1 Peter 2:4-10).

In your privileged position as a Christian serving others through healthcare, you have the single-encounter opportunity to heal a body, teach a soul, and speak to a spirit, as Jesus did. As His agent of grace and redemption, certainly you work hard to heal broken bodies and alleviate suffering, just as He did. As you do, remember that Jesus was also using His encounters with the sick to teach things with authority that people had never heard before. While you are with a hurting, suffering, or dying patient, don't neglect finding educational, hopeful, and transformative ways to teach how their physical stone can be used as a cornerstone for their future …now and into eternity.

↺ Become a Soulmate –Teach Souls

Christians in healthcare are profoundly privileged to walk in Jesus' footsteps, with the ability in a single patient encounter to heal a body, teach a soul (emotions, intellect, memories, and will), and speak to a spirit, as our Lord did. We are commissioned and empowered to do this (see Matthew 4:23-25; 9:35-10:42). The Apostle Paul, immediately after his statement on teaching souls, said, *I charge you by the Lord that this letter be read to all the brothers* (1 Thessalonians 5:27). Thus teaching souls is not optional for Christians in healthcare, or any other vocation for that matter.

What does it mean to teach a soul? Paul gives us an outline of soul-teaching:

> *And we exhort you, brothers: warn those who are irresponsible, comfort the discouraged, help the weak, be patient with everyone. See to it that no one repays evil for evil to anyone, but always pursue what is good for one another and for all.*

> 1 Thessalonians 5:14-15

Exhort is a fabulous double-edged word, meaning to counsel those who don't know what to do to do it, and admonishing those who do know what to do, but refuse to do it. Paul is exhorting us to teach souls. Here's how:

- **Warn the irresponsible. (Will)** Patient autonomy is all well and good, and we should always speak with gentleness and respect, but we must not let fear of offense prevent us from warning people that their lack of will power or their stubborn will puts them at risk, if that's their situation.

212

- **Comfort the discouraged. (Emotions)** As Christians who frequently meet with people in emotional turmoil, we should recognize and thrive in our special role of God's agents to dispense comfort, grace, and hope (2 Corinthians 1:3-11).

- **Help the weak. (Intellect)** Sometimes apparent weakness is simply a manifestation of ignorance: nobody has taught your patients how to take better care of themselves or given them the tools to do so. Remember, the knowledge you give which leads to their understanding and application becomes wisdom. *For by Wisdom your days will be many, and years will be added to your life* (Proverbs 9:11).

- **Be patient with everyone. (Memories)** God is patient with you; you live in His likeness when you extend the same patience to your patient. Don't dwell on or dredge up memories of past mistakes or failures.

- **See to it that no one repays evil for evil to anyone, but always pursue what is good for one another and for all.** Unforgiveness and anger are known to be detrimental to the soul and the body. Be discerning and address these issues with your patients if they appear to be negatively affecting their health

Teaching souls is a privilege and responsibility for Christians in healthcare. Let's be sure to ask the Holy Spirit to give us the discernment in our patient encounters to know when being a soulmate is an essential part of excellent healthcare for our patient.

ᗖ Sowing & Harvesting

In the parable about sowing the seed of the Word into the good soil of hearts ready to respond to it by faith and deeds, Jesus said the following:

> *Still others (seeds) fell on good ground and pro-*
> *duced a crop that increased 30, 60 and 100 times*
> *what was sown.' Then he said, 'Anyone who has*
> *ears to hear should listen!'...But the (seeds) sown*
> *on good ground are those who hear the word, wel-*
> *come it, and produce a crop: 30, 60 and 100 times*
> *what was sown.*
>
> Mark 4:8-9, 20

There are important principles embodied in this entire parable, but from this excerpt, allow me to simply remind each of you about two that apply to us in healthcare ministry.

The first is that there has to be good soil out there, waiting to receive the seed, or there would never be any crops to harvest. The world would starve to death, so to speak. So don't let any fear of some seed being cast on stone, or shallow or weedy soil, keep you from sowing all you can. You are not responsible for the quality of the soil. You are responsible to sow seed in whatever soil is in your path, some of which will be good. (If you are still feeling timid about what might happen if you share your faith and someone rejects it, bolster your courage and conviction by reviewing Joshua 1:9; 2 Timothy 1:7; and, 1 Peter 4:14.)

Second, in God's economy, very rare is the plant grown from seed that only bears one new seed for harvest. New plants almost always produce far more seeds for future nourishment and sowing. YOU once were a single seed germinated by faith, but now look at the opportunities God has

214

given you through healthcare to plant, say, 5 to 30 seeds each day you work!

Jesus made clear through the entire parable and its explanation that His expectation is that you will spend your life sowing with the anticipation of reaping a harvest. *"Produce a crop."* Be bold with the trust your patients give you to care for them excellently in body, soul, and spirit, the power of the Holy Spirit in you, and your conviction that God has placed you in the privileged position of being a minister of the Gospel through healthcare. Sow, sow, sow and watch God bless the harvest.

> You are not responsible for the quality of the soil. You are responsible to sow seed in whatever soil is in your path.

☙ Beware of Favoritism

How many of us remember having a teacher whom we thought had a favorite student; the one we called the teacher's pet? Maybe you had a sports coach who seemed to have one or two people he would consistently call upon while you just kept the bench warm. How did that make you feel? How did you feel towards the apparent favorites? More than that, how did it make you feel about the teacher or the coach? Did you lose respect for them?

Maybe I'm just sensitive to such things, but I've heard an idea creeping into a lot of Christian medical and dental conversations recently, and it has to do with the idea that God plays favorites. It strikes me that it is an idea that is potentially as bad for morale and our view of God and men as the earthly situation. So if I may, I want to just share a brief caution. God doesn't have favorites and those who follow Him in their medical practice shouldn't either.

> God doesn't have favorites and those who follow Him in their medical practice shouldn't either.

When God was teaching Israel about justice and equity, He warned against giving poor people any special treatment (Exodus 23:3). When teaching on family relations, He also warned against favoritism within a household. Jacob and King David would persistently suffer trouble in their homes because they didn't learn this lesson (Deuteronomy 21:15-17).

The New Testament is overflowing with declarations that God doesn't play favorites and with admonitions for the saints against having favorites in their conduct towards their fellow human beings. The Apostles Peter (Acts 10:34),

Paul (Romans 2:11, Galatians 2:6, Ephesians 6:9, Colossians 3:25, and 1 Timothy 5:21), and James (James 2:1-9, 3:17) all speak about impartiality.

The point? God does not care more for one group or class of persons, let alone individuals, than any other – not children over the elderly, poor over rich, refugee over native. Not by gender, nationality, or education does God discriminate. Scripture is very clear that God does not show favoritism, and neither should His people.

Next time you engage in a conversation or teachable moment, rather than saying "God has a special place in His heart or a special concern for…," consider saying, "I am so glad that God cares equally for all people, so that in His heart every human being is equally worthy of compassionate care." *For God so loved the whole world…*

❧ Be a Stephen in Your Workplace

I want to introduce you to a role model for our Christian healthcare. Maybe reading about this role model will embolden and encourage each of us to step out in faith and let God be part of our healthcare ministry.

In Acts 6, we are introduced to Stephen. We know little about Stephen's background except that he was likely a Messianic Jew of Hellenistic background. Yet when he does step into God's written history, he does so with a boldness and power seldom matched by any apostle or prophet. Really, he is quite amazing, since it appears that all the ministry impact he had came with believing by faith in the Gospel and learning from the apostolic teaching. This is the same source for faith and life that we all share.

Scripture says of Stephen: he was a man of good reputation, filled with the Holy Spirit, possessed wisdom, was full of grace and power, and he performed great wonders and signs before the people. In the faithful discharge of his lay duties in the Jerusalem church, he freed the apostles to preach and teach so that the spreading of God's Word flourished and the number of Christ's disciples multiplied greatly. What a reputation!

> God can take ordinary people and do extraordinary things through them if they will be devoted and make themselves available.

It might appear that Stephen was somehow unique. However, upon closer examination, Stephen is not praised for being someone special. He is praised for using the special gifts God made available to him for growth and ministering to others in a selfless and consistently dependable way. God blessed his dedication and devotion by enabling Stephen to perform wonders and signs. Stephen's life shows us that God can take ordinary people and do extraordinary things through them if they will be devoted and make themselves available to serve Him through serving others.

Application Questions

Here are a few questions for those of us who don't seem yet to be fully living up to our God-given potential to practice truly Christian healthcare.

How is your reputation? Are those who know you aware of your relationship with Jesus? Would they believe you really follow Him based on the way people see you behaving?

Do you seek to be filled with the Holy Spirit? Do you seek to let God's Spirit, not your flesh, control your life?

What's your wisdom quotient? Do you take the knowledge found in Scripture and compare it to the ways of the world so that you gain understanding? Do you then take that understanding of how God's ways are different than human ways and apply it to life, so your walk is genuinely distinct?

Can you be counted as faithful in using the gifts God has given you to dependably minister to others? Can the people around you count on you, so that they too are free to use their gifts, rather than having to cover for you?

If you are working to grow in each of these applications of Stephen's story, then there is no discernable reason why you shouldn't expect God to move in miraculous ways through you too. Marvelous things that bless God and edify people ought to be a normal part of your Christian healthcare ministry. Amen.

ҩ Another Look at Stephen

The application of Stephen's story (Acts 6-8) led us in Part 1 to a series of questions regarding our character and whether we are asking God to make us women and men of God who have a character as high as Stephen's. If we are, we should expect wondrous things to be taking place in our classrooms and practice.

> On the surface, being stoned for speaking God's truth hardly seems like a model we want to emulate.

Let's take one more look at Stephen's story. On the surface, being stoned for speaking God's truth hardly seems like a model we want to emulate. Yet there are some important things for us to grab in this difficult story that apply to us, even if we never face death for speaking publicly about Jesus.

First, standing back and looking at Stephen's situation, we see that he got into trouble with 'religious' people for speaking the truth about God. When it came time to give a defense, he didn't back away from telling God's truth. Instead, he leaned into it. Are we as steadfast when the world gets on our case for mentioning God?

Second, Stephen's defense shows that God is always moving forward in a direction He has ordained. He does so generation after generation. He has not stopped. There is a place for us as His people even now. Do we believe that, though? Do we live like we believe it?

Third, God's desires are human redemption and Christ's glory. Do we take those desires into our practices and into our classrooms? Stephen did. From a worldly viewpoint,

Stephen failed and suffered a great setback. In heaven, however, Christ stood up from His throne to encourage and welcome Stephen for his faithful work well done. Stephen's 'tragedy' became the heritage model of the Apostle Paul and the rest of us who love Jesus. Countless lives have been saved because of Stephen's bold faith. Will we be as boldly faithful and forgiving as Stephen?

As Christians in healthcare, we are uniquely privileged. We not only have the authority of God to be courageous and bold, but the authority granted by our patients to care for them. Most people desire that care to encompass body, soul, and spirit. Will we go in that authority, according to the witness of Stephen, and see wondrous things accomplished for God's glory and the redemption of humanity?

❧ Your Opportunity to Edify

Each year there are hundreds, if not thousands, of students coming to North Carolina schools to begin training for a healthcare vocation. If the enthusiastic engagement of the new students and residents at Campbell, Duke, and UNC are a reflection of the attitudes statewide, there is much about which to be excited and hopeful.

When talking with incoming and rising students, residents and fellows, two desires very quickly and prominently rise to the surface. As a fellowship of Christians in healthcare, we all have an opportunity to address both desires.

First, the new folks want and need to find a church. They want to do so in a hurry. To that end, they are very receptive to those who are excited about their church and invite new comers to join them for worship and fellowship. So put up your antennae and listen for an opportunity to help someone in transition find a welcoming church home. Maybe it will be yours!

Second, students in particular long to be in fellowship with at least one Christian healthcare provider who is more experienced than themselves. You might call it mentorship, but a better term might be mentorship-light. It includes an exchange of contact information, informal time together, maybe over a meal, and honest dialogue about medicine in general, and particularly how your Christian faith influences how you practice and lead.

Lots of second through fourth year students will be on the move though clinics and rotations all across the state. Ask the Holy Spirit to prompt you to respond to that student who might benefit from spending a little time with you. If you are faculty in a teaching setting, why not let the students know you are a believer? They may seek you out first when stress and challenges start to bear down on them.

ଛ The Life Is in the Blood

As the autumn and winter days grew shorter and colder, and as my desk/windshield/meeting time dramatically increased, my desire for warm, filling, healthy food increased. I was eating *more* hot oatmeal, whole grains, beans, fruit, etc. However, by late January, I didn't feel well at all. Lethargic, tubby, and other things, I went to see my Christian PCP.

Funny how we don't see the obvious in ourselves. But the blood tests and my observant doctor did. I had stressed, de-exercised, and carb-loaded myself into a miserable state of metabolic syndrome.

As if the Jesus of John 5:5-9 were standing in the room, Ron looked me straight in the eyes and asked, "Do you want to get healthy?" Recognizing that I too needed someone to stand beside me and help me, I answered in the affirmative. So he made some dramatic recommendations.

By faith I took his advice. Voila! In a matter of three weeks, I too picked up my mat and walked, feeling as fit as in my high school days. I am so glad to have a Christian healthcare partner who helped heal my body, taught my soul (new ways of thinking), and prayed for me, even allowing me to be accountable to him.

In Leviticus 17:10-14, we learn three things: life is found in the blood, God's plan is that the life blood is the instrument of atonement (at-one-ment), and that eating it (as the pagans did) was a sin.

How many people in healthcare routinely and reflexively turn to a blood test to guide physical or mental health diagnosis or treatment? We, too, have learned the life is in the blood. *The earthly life.*

In John 6:26-59, Jesus declared that *eternal* life is found in eating His flesh and drinking His blood. This was too shocking to believe given the people's upbringing under the Law, so many Jewish disciples fell away. But the fact remains: the blood of Jesus is effectual only if we internalize it ... by faith. *Spiritual life is in THE blood.*

As Hebrews 10:1-18 points out, the yearly practice of pouring out the blood of an animal on the altar brought annual atonement, soothing the conscience, but did not bring eternal life. Only by letting Jesus *into* our life is the shedding of His blood effectual for our eternal life and health. His blood marks the new covenant of God with humanity.

Next time you order a blood test, or review the results with your patient present, how about saying something like this:

"Ms. _____, let's have a look at your blood work. After all, as both my medical training and my Bible studies have taught me, the life is in the blood."

If your patient shows any interest in your statement, maybe asking for an explanation, you could say something like, "We know we can learn a great deal about the health of the body or issues related to the mind from examining the physical blood. What a patient's physical blood doesn't tell us though is the health of their spirit. For that we have to look to different blood."

> Only by letting Jesus into our life is the shedding of His blood effectual for our eternal life and health.

If the patient continues to be interested, expose Jesus to them. "God's Word, the Bible, has shown *me* (expose, not impose) that in order to be certain of a healthy spiritual life, I must trust in the blood of Jesus which was shed to pay for my sins. When I trust in who He is and what He did on my behalf, I am in effect letting His blood purchase my eternal health. Think of my trusting Jesus as having a voluntary transfusion, so to speak, of His perfect, sinless blood, which caused my spirit to be born again. Now I live with the resurrected Jesus in a healthy relationship forever. You can, too."

I pray this will help you leverage what so many of us do routinely into a genuine full-orbed patient care encounter.

✂ It Matters Where You Put the Stress

Have you ever had a season when every sermon or preacher or small group meeting seemed to hit on the same theme? Didn't it make you wonder if God was sending you a message to pay attention?

I've had that happen as I travel throughout our community listening to Christian healthcare practitioners. Over and over again, people expressed similar remarks about how they felt abused, misused, or deceived by a patient, co-worker, an institution, or the healthcare system in general. The sentiments were often a frustrated desire to lash out, to be heard or to exact some degree of revenge. There certainly was an air of stress among us. The critical question is what we do with the stress – where do we put it to get rid of it? Do we put it on other people and create more stress, or do we give it to God for His perfect tending?

> What do we do with the stress – where do we put it to get rid of it?

Psalm 137 is one of those psalms that speaks of community stress – practicing vocations that we love in an environment where they seem appreciated mostly for wrong or inappropriate reasons. Let's see if we can use Psalm 137 to find God's plan for where we are to put our stress.

> *By the rivers of Babylon—there we sat down and wept when we remembered Zion.*
> *2 There we hung up our lyres on the poplar trees,*
> *3 for our captors there asked us for songs,*
> *and our tormentors, for rejoicing:*
> *"Sing us one of the songs of Zion."*
> *4 How can we sing the Lord's song on foreign soil?*

227

⁵ If I forget you, Jerusalem, may my right hand forget its skill.
⁶ May my tongue stick to the roof of my mouth if I do not remember you, if I do not exalt Jerusalem as my greatest joy!
⁷ Remember, Lord, what the Edomites said that day at Jerusalem:
"Destroy it! Destroy it down to its foundations!"
⁸ Daughter Babylon, doomed to destruction, happy is the one who pays you back what you have done to us.
⁹ Happy is he who takes your little ones and dashes them against the rocks.

The captive Hebrew musicians were aliens far from their destroyed temple and former workplace in Jerusalem. The natives did not worship the Lord. Hebrew music giving glory to God may as well have been barroom ditties to the non-Jews. The musicians found themselves gathered in lament under the trees on a river bank, with their lyres – the tools of their ministry and trade – hung in trees. It could be because they had given up playing their lyres. Or it could be because they were articles of worship to God, and the only way to keep them off the ground was to hang them. Dramatic difference. Which was the more likely?

How can we sing the LORD 's song on foreign soil? (Psalm 137:4) Where we put our stress in reading makes all the difference in how we interpret the text. If we put our stress on "foreign," then this question leads us down the path of isolationism, hiding our light under a basket, and backing away from doing what God had gifted and called us to do. On the other end of the question is the word "How...?" Read with the stress put there, the psalm instantly becomes a teaching of expectant victory even in the midst of troublesome abuse, for it asks God to help us make good come of the bad.

Putting Our Stress on "How?"

- **Be Realistic** (v.1-3). We are aliens and strangers passing through. Mankind has fallen. So we need to curb our expectations for justice, common sense, and decency to be the order of the day.

- **Fix Your Mind and Ministry on God** (v.4-6). Fix your mind on the things God has done for you, is doing through you, and has in store for you. Focus ministry on serving others with the love of God.

- **Leave the Vengeance and Repayment to God** (v.7-9). No doubt these verses seem brutal to our delicate sensibilities. Nevertheless, if God is who He says He is and if He is worthy of our reverent fear, then we must submit to His command and let Him mete out justice. We cannot judge another person's heart, but He can. He can discern the difference between someone hurting us by error or oversight, or deliberately abusing us.

- **Finally, Cast Your Cares on Him, Coming to Him with Your Burdens.** The most misused and abused person was Jesus. His answer to stress was always the same: pray. If prayer, rather than quitting or exacting retribution, was our Lord's solution to life's stresses, then isn't it a good idea to follow Him in putting our emphasis on prayer too?

ぞ We Need Art Restorers

Recently, I visited eight houses of worship for Roman Catholics, Lutherans, Evangelicals, and Russian Orthodox worshipers in the Rhine region of Germany. The buildings ranged in age from the early 1200s to the late 1800s. All featured stone, wood, and glass as key building materials, though the materials were fitted together in a variety of layouts and proportions, sort of like early and very large Lego sets. Almost all the buildings had undergone varying degrees of restoration due to age, wear, or war.

In the early mornings before touring, I sat down to read through Dr. John Wyatt's *Matters of Life and Death* (InterVarsity Press, Nottingham, 2009). Featured prominently in Dr. Wyatt's discussion of Christian faith and praxis in the modern age of medicine and bioethics is a similar analogy to buildings. He asks whether human beings are like Lego sets, collections of interchangeable and replaceable parts without an internal, natural order and without a "single purpose for which the kit is intended by its designers" (pg. 97). Or, are humans the product of a master artist, created with an intended natural, internal order for a unified purpose?

If the former is the worldview of society, philosophers, or secular healthcare providers, then when a person becomes aged, worn, or broken, medicine can now add or subtract parts to make something new or different. Or if that is too costly or complicated, medicine can quietly dismiss the person as no longer useful. Think of it this way: if the world's tallest church, built in the 14th century at Ulm, needed repair, why not go all the way and remodel it to look like the 21st century stainless steel and triple-pane green glass of the Audi Museum Mobile in Ingolstadt just down the tracks? Another option would be to tear it down.

230

If the latter worldview is the case, then when a masterpiece of God's creation in His image and likeness becomes aged, worn, or damaged, the Christian practitioner will serve as a skilled art restorer, doing a restoration of the artist's creation to its original design and intended purpose, to the highest degree possible.

This concept of restoration is very much what King David was looking for spiritually in his penitent appeal to God in Psalm 51. So whether you are healing bodies, teaching souls, or speaking to spirits, be an art restorer.

❧ Sharing a Good Report

There is no doubt that most of us as Christian healthcare providers feel a calling to share the love and eternal life Jesus offers with our patients. Yet most of us don't or rarely do. I've observed in numerous conversations that most folks are 'under-discipled' in this area. Several opportunities to do small group 10-minute teachings have opened many eyes to the possibilities in our settings for sharing Jesus in a manner tailored to our particular kind of practice.

Let me give you an example of such training and a good report that happened recently. I met with a small group of dental students and shared a dentist-tailored 10-minute teaching. Embedded in that was the fact that God didn't design creation with pain from decay or disease and death, but it came with sin. Yet God still cares about these things and died for our sins so that one day we won't have to experience sin, pain, or death. In the meantime, God cares about our pain and fears. Additionally, the students were encouraged to expect to be used as part of a divine appointment every day. Be on the lookout for the person to whom the Holy Spirit will lead you to speak love and truth.

> Be on the lookout for the person to whom the Holy Spirit will lead you to speak love and truth.

In less than six hours, I received this text message from one of the students, which I have permission to share with you. Remember, it's a text message, so it is necessarily an abbreviated record of a conversation. "I got to share the Lord with a patient just testifying that her being in pain was not the Lord's will for her. He must love us because He laid down His life on the cross for us, and that there would not have to be any tooth extractions in heaven!"

To God be the glory! Rejoice with this student who got to share God's love in a wonderful way with someone who needed to hear it. If you are willing to learn, you can experience the same kind of joy this student did. Are you willing and ready to learn?

᷒ Approved Words & Godless Chatter

The Apostle Paul took teaching, learning, and application very seriously:

> *Do your best to present yourself to God as one approved, a workman who does not need to be ashamed and who correctly handles the Word of truth. Avoid godless chatter, because those who indulge in it will become more and more ungodly.*
>
> 2 Timothy 2:15-16, NIV

There are only so many hours left in our lives before we have to give an account of what we did with the talents we were given. Most of us are very good at learning about and applying our medical knowledge. Certainly there will be temporal rewards and gratification for being a good workman in our field. However, even our best craftsmanship is only temporary; our patients will die one day.

Paul called on Timothy, and by extension us, to be skilled at handling the Word of God, which is the only skill we are called to use that has eternal durability. It will not return void. It is the only way for saving faith to enter anyone's life.

Basketball tournaments, spring weather, gloating on our kids – even discussing the latest medical breakthroughs – are all interesting. But, in a sense, they are 'godless,' unless you are deliberate about inserting the Word of God into the conversation. People who are your neighbors walk away from a conversation with you a few minutes older and a few minutes further from eternal life, if you don't love these neighbors by exposing Jesus to them.

Be a workman approved, avoiding godless chatter.

❧ Don't Harm the Oil & the Wine

My vocation is serving the Christian healthcare community, where I've often mentioned that Christians in healthcare are not superior, but they are uniquely privileged to walk in the footsteps of Jesus. As you are about to discover, even in terrible times of tribulation, it seems Jesus has a special plan for Christians in healthcare.

Bible Background

In the Book of Revelation, when Jesus opened the third seal of the scroll, John saw this vision.

> *And I looked, and there was a black horse. The horseman on it had a balance scale in his hand. Then I heard something like a voice among the four living creatures say, "A quart of wheat for a denarius, and three quarts of barley for a denarius — but do not harm the olive oil and the wine.*

Revelation 6:5b-6

Our Lord's interpretation of the four horsemen, found in Matthew 24:4-8, tells us this horseman represents famine, apparently caused by either a failure in growth of raw foods or in food production/distribution. This famine follows counterfeit prophets, then global warfare, and precedes a continuation of these plus the addition of disease and disaster. Yet the oil and wine are to be preserved. Why?

First, for the nation of Israel, the Lord considered oil and wine as essential elements of worship. Unlike the other elements of worship such as grain or livestock, olive trees and grape vines were the only two *perennial* elements. This speaks of how even in times of tribulation, there will be a remnant of elect among whom worship will not end.

Second, who was it that Jesus said in Luke 10:25-37 would inherit eternal life? The one who completely loved God and neighbor. How did the good Samaritan demonstrate those loves? When he came upon a wounded man who had been brutally abused and then neglected, He poured out in a loving and sacrificial way the perennial elements of worship which also happened to be the medicinally cleansing, soothing, and sealing oil and wine!

Application

As Jesus went on to say later in Matthew 24:36-44, nobody knows when these terrible times of tribulation will come. Maybe we will be alive. Maybe it will be the future generations of Christians in healthcare in whom we invest our time and teaching. Either way, there are two important applications for how we practice healthcare as Christians.

First, it seems obvious that the Lord sees a special role for Christians in healthcare. There is no separating our living a life of worship and witness from our medical ministry to our neighbors. Regardless of the degree of tribulation, those of us with this calling cannot rightly decouple our faith and practice.

Second, we don't know when Christ is going to start opening the scroll, but He has called us to keep watch and daily be about the Master's business. There is already plenty of tribulation going around – we don't need to wait for some future time. Let's be faithful today and every day to walk in our Lord's footsteps, sharing our worship as an integral part of our medical ministry.

In a wonderfully poetic and yet realistic play on words, the prophet Malachi speaks of the tumultuous Day of the Lord, when the sun will no longer shine:

But to you who fear My name the Sun of Right-
eousness shall arise with healing in His wings;
and you shall go out and grow fat like stall-fed
calves.

Malachi 4:2; NKJV

May you see your vocation as a Christian in healthcare as
an opportunity to walk in the footsteps of the Sun of Righteousness, teaching the fear of the Lord, and offering healing
as a perennial act of worship.

❧ Keeping Relevant

I don't have to tell most of you that the Apostle Peter commands us to be ready to give an explanation for the hope we have (1 Peter 3:15). Nor do I need to remind you that the Apostle Paul called the Word of God "the sword of the Spirit" (Ephesians 6:17). Finally, you are already probably aware that Jesus promised that the Spirit would remind the disciples what to say when people confronted them and asked them questions (John 14:26). Most of us know these things. Yet, based upon the testimony of many, many Christians in healthcare, all too often we finish a day of classes or patient care with a little nagging sense we weren't ready, did not see the Holy Spirit wield His sword, and didn't know what to say to that certain person with whom we came in contact. Why? Allow me to share my observations. Hopefully they will help you.

First, I used to not begin every day believing that God wanted to use me and daily had a divine appointment waiting for me. I was mistaken. I've learned He wants to use me every day. Every day is a gift from God to be used for His glory, so of course He wants to use me. I just had to start expecting Him to and the blinders to my divine appointments fell away.

> I meditate on your precepts and consider your ways. I delight in your decrees. I will not neglect your word.
>
> Psalm 119:15-16

Second, I let every excuse keep me from reading or listening to God's Word daily. No reading, no listening? No swords stored up in the armory of my mind for the Holy

Spirit to draw out. If I am not putting any of God's Word into my mind, *then what exactly is it the Holy Spirit is going to remind me of?* Am I supposed to whip out John 3:16 – the only sword I've put in my armory in the last number of months or years – and trust it is the right sword for any and every type of situation I may face or every need my patients or peers have?

Practical Tips

Are you an eye doc? Immerse yourself in Gospel passages where Jesus spoke about sight, seeing, or darkness and light. How did He heal the blind, physically and spiritually? Are you a PT/OT? How did Jesus engage the lame and the crippled? Are you a dentist? How does Jesus address those with fear in their lives? Do you deal with souls? What does Jesus say to those afflicted with guilt or issues of forgiveness? Are you an anesthesiologist? What does Jesus have to say to those who need rest? Are you an RN or PA involved in pediatrics and/or family medicine? Oh, the examples of children and parents coming to Christ from which you can mine God's riches! The examples go on and on across the entire spectrum of Christian healthcare practices.

Once you have hidden these historic accounts away in your mind and heart for the Holy Spirit to draw on, then listen for the Holy Spirit to prompt you. Share the account appropriate for your situation with your patient in a winsome way. Don't lecture, but tell the story and give a personal testimony of what moved, touched, or changed YOU when YOU read it. How did it make you love or appreciate God in a greater way? You can't make arbitrary promises of healing, but, based on these accounts, you can assure your patients or peers that God knows and cares about them in body, soul, and spirit.

It will be a rare case when someone will argue with you about your own story. You are much more likely to be asked where that story can be found in the Bible so they can read it for themselves. If you are really on your game expecting a divine appointment, you'll have a giveaway Bible in one of your scrub pockets or an exam room drawer. Mark the story for them and give it away – for it certainly will not return void but will accomplish the purpose for which God sent it (Isaiah 55:10-11).

✑ Keeping Promises

Being honest, you realize that you can't promise patients a certain outcome. That's why everyone has to sign an informed consent document. However, God does keep all of His promises. Jesus repeatedly promised that even though He would die, He would rise to life again on the third day. He declared He had the Father's authority to lay down His life and to take it up again. He said that those who believed in Him, even though they die would never die, not ever. He was making some big-time promises about having life more abundantly and life eternally. He kept making these pronouncements in the context of going throughout the land healing, teaching, and preaching.

The resurrection is the evidence that you can bank on Jesus' promises. You have solid, tangible, verified evidence that Jesus wasn't boasting, bragging, or offering what He wasn't able to deliver. The resurrection is proof that

> God does keep all of His promises.

when Jesus offers to cure believers forevermore of all physical and soulish diseases and spiritual death, He can and will do it. By faith in Him people become new creations now and will rise in new, imperishable, incorruptible, glorified bodies, souls, and spirits.

Admitting you can't make promises also gives you an opportunity to share Jesus with your patients. You can say how glad you are that you know someone who *can* make promises and has proven He can and will keep them. Jesus wasn't boasting or bragging when He made His promises. He proved them. That's why you celebrate and trust Him.

ᔥ The Rain of God

When it comes to weather, we don't always understand why some people must suffer record heat while others endure a deluge. What we do know is that God is good, that He authored both heat and rain for a beneficial purpose, and that He often uses physical elements like rain to teach us important spiritual lessons. Rain is a favorite teaching tool of the Holy Spirit, as shown in this passage from Isaiah.

> *⁶ Seek the LORD while He may be found;*
> *call to Him while He is near.*
> *⁷ Let the wicked one abandon his way, and the sinful one his thoughts; let him return to the LORD, so He may have compassion on him, and to our God, for He will freely forgive.*
> *⁸ "For My thoughts are not your thoughts,*
> *and your ways are not My ways."*
>
> *This is the LORD 's declaration.*
>
> *⁹ "For as heaven is higher than earth, so My ways are higher than your ways, and My thoughts than your thoughts.*
> *¹⁰ For just as rain and snow fall from heaven, and do not return there without saturating the earth, and making it germinate and sprout, and providing seed to sow and food to eat,*
> *¹¹ so My word that comes from My mouth will not return to Me empty, but it will accomplish what I please, and will prosper in what I send it to do."*
> *¹² You will indeed go out with joy and be peacefully guided;*
> *the mountains and the hills will break into singing before you, and all the trees of the field will clap their hands.*

[13] Instead of the thornbush, a cypress will come up,
and instead of the brier, a myrtle will come up;
it will make a name for the LORD as an everlasting
sign that will not be destroyed.

Isaiah 55:6-13

Application

First, in verses 10-11, God links rain, and the manifold goodness it was designed to bring, to His Word. Rain doesn't fall willy-nilly; God's Word isn't idle chatter.

Second, the context of verses 6-9 tells us that as rain has a powerful ability to wash away dirt and filth, so too does God's Word wash away the guilty stains of sin. God is desirous of our cleansing and generous with the agents He provides to effect it.

Third, as falling rain today serves as a promise of a green future, God's Word – as it falls on our ears – gives a promise of a flourishing eternal life. While this is good news for us, it is most certainly also for God's glorious renown.

As you engage in numerous conversations about the weather, as you surely will, may they be reminders to you that you have the privilege of sprinkling the conversation with the truth that God gave rain for our physical good and He desires to pour spiritual rain into our lives as well.

∂ Are You a Snow Blower?

Winter comes and snow can pile up. When it does, it gets me thinking about how we can parlay this weather into an opportunity to expose the love of God to our patients who will surely be open to discussing snow for the next few weeks. We can become snow blowers!

The Prophet Isaiah, speaking for God at the beginning and near the end of his book, mentioned the image of snow. The first passage reads,

> *"Come, let us discuss this," says the LORD.*
> *"Though your sins are like scarlet, they will be as*
> *white as snow; though they are as red as crimson,*
> *they will be like wool. If you are willing and obe-*
> *dient, you will eat the good things of the land."*
>
> Isaiah 1:18-19

God calls people to Himself through reason, not coercion. He promises complete forgiveness of sin and its eternal consequences. True to His nature, which we all reflect, He allows us to make a choice to respond or reject His call to have a blessed relationship with Him.

Here's some suggestions on how to use this passage to become a snow blower.

- Mention how all the snowfall reminded YOU of this passage.

- Comment how YOU found great comfort in knowing God wanted a relationship with YOU and was willing to give YOU an opportunity to reason with Him about what that meant.

244

- Reveal that YOU have found God's call reasonable and have accepted it.

- Declare YOU are the recipient of many "good things of the land" by trusting God.

Notice you are only telling YOUR story, exposing God's love. Never are you imposing God on anyone. You are just blowing His snow of cleansing.

In the following passage from Isaiah there are many opportunities to expose the love of God, using the snow motif again, to a patient who expresses an interest to learn more. You can continue to be a snow blower for God.

> *Seek the LORD while He may be found; call to Him while He is near. Let the wicked one abandon his way and the sinful one his thoughts; let him return to the LORD, so He may have compassion on him, and to our God, for He will freely forgive. For My thoughts are not your thoughts, and your ways are not My ways. This is the LORD's declaration.*
>
> *For as heaven is higher than earth, so My ways are higher than your ways, and My thoughts than your thoughts. For just as rain and snow fall from heaven and do not return there without saturating the earth and making it germinate and sprout, and providing seed to sow and food to eat, so My word that comes from My mouth will not return to Me empty, but it will accomplish what I please and will prosper in what I send it to do.*
>
> Isaiah 55:6-11

God says there is an invitation to seek Him and be completely, compassionately forgiven for our offenses against Him. At first we may not understand all that this call to be

245

forgiven means. Understanding grows as we spend time in His Word. Trusting God means He will guide us in peace. He is not at war with us, as we were with Him. God will give purpose to the life that has set its soul on following Him. NOBODY is excluded from God's call. NOBODY – no matter what they have done in the past and how messed up they seem now. God will join all of His children, regardless of their past, into one new humanity, complete in Jesus Christ (Ephesians 2:11-22).

Your patients will be eager to talk snow in the next few weeks. Will you transform your encounter with them from a temporary one to an eternally significant one by becoming a snow blower for God?

ᔕ Spiritual History: Why Take One?

From various conversations with Christian health care students and practitioners, I've observed we have an intellectual knowledge that we are salt and light, as Jesus declared. However, many of us also have a low-grade sense of guilt because in our professional arenas we shy away from outright salting and lighting. While there are many reasons why Christians shy away, I want to focus on just one to encourage you. That reason is a mistaken belief that faith and/or spirituality (*seeking someone or something sacred*) has no place in medical ministry. We have been trained professionally or culturally to accept that when a patient presents with a physical or mental need, the practitioner is acting out of scientific bounds by introducing faith or spirituality into the care space.

Research shows there are significant benefits to the patient when the healthcare practitioner introduces spirituality and/or faith into the care plan. In fact, the research is so clear on this that the Joint Commission mandates that hospitals respect patients' beliefs and accommodate their right to religious and spiritual services (Joint Commission Standard: *The Hospital Respects, Protects, and Promotes Patient Rights*; RI.01.01.01, EP6, EP9). But how will this happen unless somebody takes a Spiritual

> Research shows there are significant benefits to the patient when the healthcare practitioner introduces spirituality and/or faith into the care plan.

Assessment? QED, the argument that "the system" rejects introducing the issue of faith and/or spirituality into the care space, or taking a spiritual history, is disproved.

But what about the fear that many patients may in some way be offended? Dr. Harold G. Koenig, in his book *Spirituality in Patient Care* (West Conshohocken, PA; Templeton Press; 2nd ed.; 2007; pp16-18), does a nice job of summarizing medical research showing that the majority of patients *want* and *increase their trust in* practitioners who take spirituality into account.

One way to reduce any risk of offense is to be proactive. Let the patient know in advance that you routinely take a Spiritual Assessment as part of your HPI or new patient screening. Borrowing again from Dr. Koenig, here is a sample of proactive information you could give to your patients or post on your workspace wall. I've adapted it to be a bit less 'clinical.'

We Care for The Whole Patient

In an effort to provide you with the best possible care, and as part of getting to know you, members of our healthcare team routinely include a Spiritual Assessment as part of your examination.

The questions are few, brief, and non-judgmental.

You can't give a 'wrong' answer.

Why we consider a Spiritual Assessment essential to excellent patient care:

1. The majority of patients consider themselves spiritual beings and want care team members to acknowledge and respect that in their care.

2. Spiritual considerations have been scientifically shown to impact health outcomes. We want to know how they may or may not help in your treatment.

3. Matters of religion may influence which kinds of treatments are or are not acceptable to you. We want to discuss, document, and respect your preferences.

4. Your or your family's faith may have a great role in dealing with medical or emotional issues. We want to support positive faith influences. If you request or consent to it, this may include care team members praying for or with you.

5. If you are hospitalized or home-bound, you may have less contact with your faith community. Our care team wants to provide what support we can to fill that gap.

6. If need be and with your permission, we may want to contact your spiritual shepherd to make him or her aware of how your faith community might help in your care.

7. We value every person as made in the image and likeness of God, and thus we want to recognize and care for the whole you: body, soul (*emotion, intellect, memories, and will*), and spirit (*the desire for and ability to connect with the sacred*).

᎒ Spiritual History Taking

Taking a quality
spiritual history
is good medicine.

Having established that taking a spiritual history is appropriate and important, and that there is a way to broach the subject with sensitive, supportive pre-work, now it is time to take the spiritual history. Here are some suggestions.

Situation One: "I want a quick way to take a patient's spiritual temperature."

Bob Mason at Medical Strategic Network suggested a single question which takes the temperature. It is not a spiritual history in itself, but it will lead to the patient giving you clues about further questions to ask. The question is, "Do you feel that prayer could be an important part of your treatment program?"

Situation Two: "I want a simple pneumonic for taking a good spiritual history I can chart and others will understand."

Walt Larrimore, MD, along with Wm. Peele, DMin in their *Grace Prescriptions* course, offer a pneumonic called the LORD's LAP. I've taken the liberty of modifying it slightly. I use GOD's LAP. The bullets below each question of the pneumonic suggest important follow-up information to be charted from the patient's responses.

G: Are <u>God</u>, religion, or spirituality important to you?

- Yes, No, or Sort of. Chart their response.
- If 'sort of,' probe. Be sure to ask the LAP questions.

O: How do <u>other</u> people support your faith, religion, or spirituality?

- What religious or spiritual community do they identify with?
- Do they have a spiritual shepherd, such as a pastor, rabbi, or imam?

D's: What may I/we <u>do</u> to care for you spiritually?

- Are there specific medical do's or don'ts? Blood, dress, gender?
- Would the patient object to prayer as part of care?
- Would the patient like counsel? Chaplain service?
- Who in the patient's faith community may you contact if need be?

Peer-reviewed research has shown that the two-year mortality rate for patients recently discharged from the hospital is 16% to 28% higher for patients who answer "Yes" to at least one of the LAP questions. Addressing the issues raised by asking them is good medicine! The bullets following the questions give you a starting place for talking about how you understand their feelings, but the Bible says God has a different perspective. (Note: Christians, Jews, Muslims, and many polytheistic systems all recognize the Old Testament as sacred Scripture.)

L: Do you feel you are ill because God does not <u>love</u> you? (-22%)

- Exodus 34:6-7a; Psalm 145:14-17; Ezekiel 18:31-32 and 33:11; Lamentations 3:31-33
- Romans 5:8; John 3:14-18; 1 John 4:9-10; Luke 15:1-24

A: Do you feel you are ill because God has <u>abandoned</u> you? (-28%)

- Deuteronomy 31:6, 8; Isaiah 41:17; Isaiah 42:16
- Luke 15:1-24; Hebrews 13:5

P: Do you feel you are ill because God is <u>punishing</u> you? (-16%)

- Ezekiel 18 and 33:1-20
- 1 Peter 1:18-20; 1 John 2:2; 1 John 1:8-10

Are you afraid taking the spiritual history might take too long? Shouldn't you really be asking, "How long will eternity be for this person God loves, and why can't I use the time I have to expose Jesus to him/her?"

Are you afraid that under financial pressures, you can't 'afford' to take a good spiritual history and discover the patient is having a religious struggle? Never fear! You can be reimbursed for the time it takes to discover it and offer good counsel or a chaplaincy referral. Add the ICD-9 code V62.89 or ICD-10 code Z65.8 to your chart.

Taking a quality spiritual history is good medicine. Since excellence in your practice is a basic expectation of Christian healthcare, then you really don't have a good excuse for not taking one if the patient is open to it.

⌘ Only the Doctor Is with Me

Would you please forgive me for being personal? These thoughts come from an experienced heart.

My first wife Sandy went to heaven due to a gynecological cancer. On one hand, it broke her mother's heart. On the other, Sandy made a transformative impression on her mom's faith by reassuring her mom she was at peace knowing she would soon be in heaven with Jesus. Sandy's mom, Marge, later developed a terminal gynecological cancer of her own. When I spoke with Marge right after her diagnosis, the first thing she said to me was to quote Sandy's hope in Jesus and claim it for hers too. Hallelujah!

As soon as I found out, I confess I flashed back to a very difficult part of Sandy's illness for me, especially as a Christian involved in healthcare. I felt the healthcare providers 'abandoned' Sandy once they had done all they could from an earthly perspective. That's not a new feeling. When the Apostle Paul was about to enter God's presence, too, he declared his confidence in Christ and his soon-coming rewards. Then Paul expressed the same sense of abandonment by men at his end (2 Timothy 4:6-18).

But Paul gave us one ray of hope, and that ray shines light on how you should think about your practice ministry to the dying. Paul said to Timothy, *"Only* [Dr.] *Luke is with me."* When everyone else was busy with their own lives, on assignment, cowardly, or cruel, Doctor Luke stuck with Paul in his end time.

"But," you say, "I can't be everywhere for everyone." True enough. But Jesus can. Have you used your trusted and unique relationship with your patient who is about to embark on a transformational and eternal journey to introduce her or him to Jesus the Great Physician? Paul knew Christ Jesus faithfully stuck with him. As believers, Sandy and I knew God was with us and wouldn't forsake us.

Still, we felt abandoned. Why? Because God created us for community and mutual support. As John Wyatt, MD notes in *Matters of Life and Death* (InterVarsity Press, Nottingham, 2009), we are born into a community with parents to care for us, we grow to be parents caring for our own new community, and as we grow older and frail, we again need to be in a community of caregivers. God's plan is for loving humans to care for and about one another in their time of suffering or frailty. When those we count on to care for us, to understand our suffering, and to have our best interest at heart stop communicating with us, we feel abandoned.

No doubt you are incredibly busy. Some of you will see hundreds of terminal patients each year. So what can you do to preclude your patient feeling abandoned by you? Here are three suggestions that take little time or effort. They may make an eternal difference.

> God's plan is for loving humans to care for and about one another in their time of suffering or frailty.

First, within 48 hours of giving someone a serious or terminal diagnosis, call your patient at home. If you do this at the end of your workday, you can tell them you are on the way home to your family but paused to check on them. They will understand you don't have much time. They will, however, be deeply moved by your personal contact. Tell them you are praying for them and offer to pray with them on the phone.

Second, have your staff help you get a greeting card to them within two weeks, and once a month thereafter. Two to three thoughtful sentences are all you need to write. But they will be received with deep gratitude.

Third, if you enroll someone in a hospice program, don't stop communicating and advocating for your patient, thinking that's someone else's job now. The patient still thinks of *you* as their doctor who cares. Tell your patient that if they don't feel they are getting the support they need, from hospice or elsewhere, they can call you. You have to make that known to your 'gatekeepers' too.

The Holy Spirit made a point of preserving Paul's comment, *"Only* [Dr.] *Luke is with me."* If He thinks that observation is important enough to pass down through the millennia to the saints, shouldn't we take heed and respond?

❧ Are You Listening?

The one who gives an answer before he listens —
this is foolishness and disgrace for him.

Proverbs 18:13

Rachel (not her real name) is a wonderful woman of God. She's articulate, thoughtful, and respectful of others. She's also been dealt a hand of bad genes, so her body wars with the wishes of her soul and spirit to serve God. RA, IDDM, neuropathy, cellulitis, and allergies to almost all known antibiotics, have landed her in the hospital for more than one month out of the last six, and in surgery five times. God pours His Spirit into her to help her cope. She's an inspiration to family and friends for her faith and trust that God will never leave or forsake her and is in these challenges. He hears and answers her prayers for grace and strength.

Rachel will testify, however, that listening seems a vanishing skill among healthcare practitioners. Over 30 years of medical challenges, some doctors stand out as least likely to listen well, not believing a patient can have so many issues or allergies. The result: nosocomial anaphylactic reactions from intentional administration of drugs on her allergy list. She's had so many she has PTSD and fears hospitalization. Add in the Death on Demand movement, and dread of an unfamiliar doctor deciding for her that her life is not worth living because of all of her health issues, and it's a terrible cocktail

> You should also strive to be as good at listening to your patients as God is at listening to those who pray to Him.

256

of psychological trauma for someone who just wants compassionate, understanding help.

How are your listening skills? Are you quick to listen and slow to speak, or has the quickening pace of healthcare demands and patient encounters dulled your hearing? Are you on the verge of surrendering your detective, problem-solving teamwork in order to become a mere technician or mechanic? Of course not every patient is as educated about her health as Rachel, or as in tune with her body. But *you'll have to listen to each person to discover* those who are able to cooperate with you in their care. Maybe someday Rachel will meet the issue which will end her mortal life. Even then though, knowing a listening practitioner stood beside her will be a comfort.

As a Christian in healthcare, you have the opportunity to walk in the very footsteps of Jesus, healing bodies, teaching souls, and speaking to spirits. You should also strive to be as good at listening to your patients as God is at listening to those who pray to Him. After all, you may in fact be the agent of grace and strength Rachel's been praying for.

About the Author

From 1984 to 1991, Paul Gerritson served in the US Air Force and at the Defense Intelligence Agency. His self-initiated research on countering mobile ballistic missile threats through creative detection led to his receipt of the National Foreign Intelligence Medal of Achievement from the Director of Central Intelligence, the US Air Force Medal of Achievement, and recognition by the Director of DIA for Meritorious Service during Operation Desert Storm.

From 1992-2005, he served as a 911 and Critical Care Paramedic and EMS Operations Director in New Mexico. He attended Wayland Baptist University and Golden Gate Baptist Theological Seminary where he earned his Master of Divinity. He pastored three congregations from 2004-2012.

Currently, Paul is the Area Director-Pastor for the Triangle Christian Medical & Dental Associations in the Raleigh, Durham, and Chapel Hill area. His life journey has equipped him to fulfill His passion: teaching those in all aspects of healthcare to use their privileged position to glorify God and serve humanity by keeping faith at the core of their practice.

Paul lives in Durham, North Carolina with his wife Judy. They enjoy cycling, tennis, and travel.